Plant Power

The essential plant food guide to enrich your health

Professor Luigi Fontana
MD, PHD, FRACP
Scientific Director, Charles Perkins Centre Royal Prince Alfred Clinic
Director, Health for Life Research and Clinical Program, University of Sydney

Marzio Lanzini
Recipe co-development and Photography

Hardie Grant

BOOKS

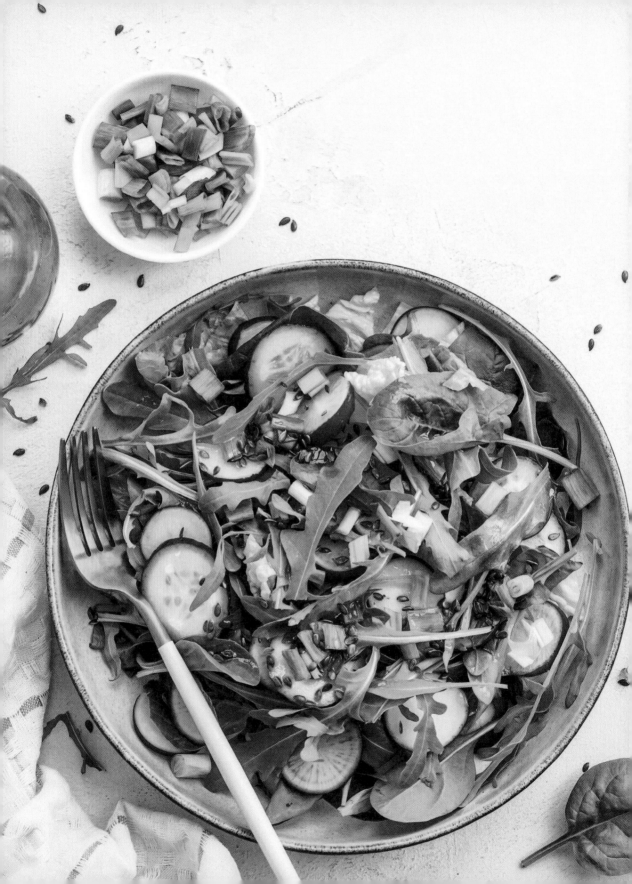

contents

foreword

The primary aim of this new book is to serve as a practical guide that brings together the latest scientific insights into healthy eating and longevity, specifically for individuals who are eager to adopt more balanced and nourishing plant-centric diets. In my clinical practice, I frequently meet patients who assume that simply removing meat from their diet will naturally result in better health. However, the truth is that achieving a well-rounded, nutritious diet requires much more than just the exclusion of meat or all animal products. It involves a thoughtful approach to meal planning that ensures all essential nutrients are adequately provided.

Many individuals who switch to vegetarian or vegan diets for ethical, environmental, religious or philosophical reasons often replace animal products with refined and processed foods, which can lead to malnutrition and increase the risk of type 2 diabetes, cardiovascular diseases, haemorrhagic stroke, bone fractures, and possibly cancer. To address these concerns, I collaborated with my esteemed colleague and friend, Professor Walter Willett, the former Chair of the Department of Nutrition at Harvard University. Together, we were tasked with reviewing the vast body of literature on the benefits and potential risks associated with vegetarian and vegan diets. Our findings were recently published in the highly regarded *European Heart Journal*. This book builds on that research, offering readers not just insights but practical tools and recipes to help them adopt healthier eating habits.

The concepts presented in this book are extensions of the theoretical groundwork laid in my earlier work, *The Path to Longevity*, published in 2020. That book provided an extensive exploration of various interventions and mechanisms that contribute to overall wellbeing – encompassing physical, metabolic, mental, emotional and spiritual health. It aimed to weave together traditional wisdom and contemporary scientific developments, presenting a comprehensive approach to health promotion, disease prevention, and achieving a longer, healthier life.

Over the years, I've received countless enquiries from my patients, friends, students and followers who are eager to learn about the best foods to eat and the most effective ways to prepare them. My hope is that this book will not only satisfy their curiosity but also equip them with the recipes and knowledge they need to make nutritious meals a part of their daily routine. For those who have found my previous books or scientific articles to be too dense or complex, this practical guide – alongside my earlier publication, *Manual of Healthy Longevity and Wellbeing* – offers straightforward and holistic strategies for living a long, vibrant life.

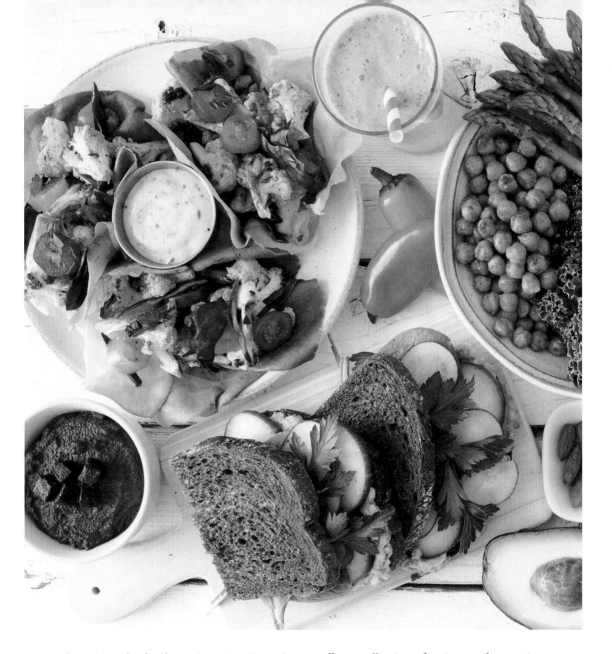

In writing this book, my intention is not just to offer a collection of recipes or dietary tips but to empower you with a deeper understanding of how food choices influence your health and longevity. This book is an invitation to explore the profound connection between what we eat and how we live, aiming to inspire you to make choices that nurture not only your body but also your mind and spirit.

Let this book be your companion on the journey to a healthier, more fulfilled life. With the right knowledge and tools, we can all take meaningful steps toward achieving longevity and wellness in a way that is both practical and sustainable.

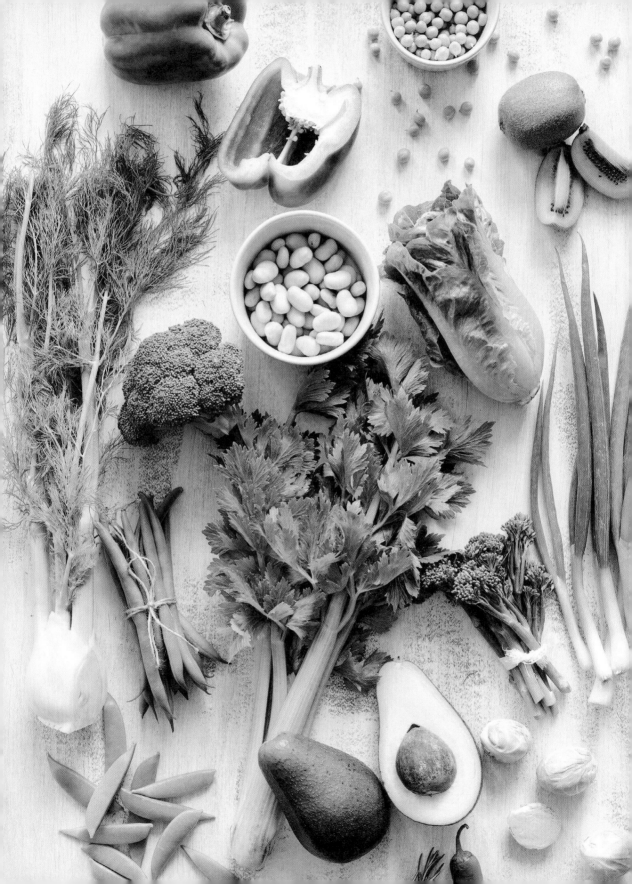

to be, or not to be vegetarian, that is the dilemma

Ask a room full of people to raise their hands if they eat a vegetarian or vegan diet, if not all of the week, then a part of the week, and some will do so. Then ask them if they believe that eating a vegetarian or vegan diet will make them healthier; the majority will raise their hands.

It's happening right across the western world. More people are turning away from meat-centric diets and incorporating more plant foods. Some are choosing to become vegetarians or vegans, the latter abstaining from all animal products, even honey. In 2023, the Statista research department published data from 2019 showing that 42 per cent of Australians are choosing to eat less meat or none at all: 10 per cent identified themselves as vegan or vegetarian, 12 per cent as a meat-reducer and 20 per cent as flexitarian. Similarly, a comprehensive 2018 Ipsos Mori poll conducted across 28 countries found that 5 per cent of respondents identified as vegetarian, 3 per cent as vegan, and 3 per cent as pescetarian, with these numbers varying significantly by country. Interestingly, younger individuals are more likely to follow these dietary choices; in the 2018 Ipsos survey, 6 per cent of those under 35 identified as vegetarians, compared to 3 per cent of those over 35.

Anecdotally, people reduce or eliminate meat from their diets for a variety of reasons. Long-term vegetarians and vegans often cite animal welfare as a key motivation. Others are influenced by social initiatives like Meat Free Monday and Veganuary, which encourage short-term adoption of vegetarian or vegan diets. Some individuals opt for vegetarian meals, even part-time, due to economic considerations, especially amid rising living costs. Younger adults, in particular, may choose vegetarian meals for easier weight management. Then there are those who've chosen to go plant-heavy because of the perceived health benefits, both for themselves and for the planet. Regardless of the extent of their dietary change, however, most people agree that eating less meat is healthier, whether they do so one day a week or every day.

Whatever someone's reason for adopting a plant-rich diet, it's clear that this is more than just a fad. There are different types of plant-focused diets, but vegan (100 per cent plant-based), lacto-ovo vegetarian (plant-centric except for the addition of dairy products and/or eggs when animals are not harmed), and pesco-vegetarian or pescatarian (plant-powered with fish and seafood, with or without eggs and dairy) are some of the most common. All vegetarian diets exclude meat – such as beef, pork, lamb, venison and chicken – as well as related meat products. In contrast, flexitarian diets emphasise plant-rich foods but allow for occasional consumption of meat and other animal products.

The problem

Many people assume that removing meat from their diet will automatically enhance their health. However, achieving a balanced and nutritious diet requires more than just cutting out meat. Often, individuals embracing vegetarian diets tend to replace meat or other animal products with foods high in refined carbohydrates, fats and salt, such as white bread, frozen pizza, instant noodles, canned soups, pre-packaged meals, pastries, cakes, cookies, French fries, chips, plant-based meat substitutes and sugary beverages.

These products are typically loaded with empty calories that promote obesity, particularly from added sugars or high-fructose corn syrup, saturated (butter, cream, coconut and palm kernel) and partially hydrogenated fats. Oils that become solid at room temperature are particularly high in saturated fats. They are always low in dietary fibre, antioxidant vitamins, minerals, trace elements and beneficial phytochemicals. Additionally, these foods may contain potentially harmful substances, including acrylamide, heterocyclic amines and polycyclic aromatic hydrocarbons, which are known to be carcinogenic. They may also contain various food additives, such as titanium dioxide (used as a whitening agent), talc and carbon black.

Multiple scientific studies indicate that people

consuming vegetarian diets high in processed and ultra-processed foods and sweetened sodas have a higher risk of diabetes, coronary heart disease and increased cardiovascular mortality than people consuming healthy flexitarian diets. Additionally, these 'unhealthy' vegetarian diets may contribute to cancer development by causing insulin resistance and other pro-inflammatory and hormonal changes, which can lead to uncontrolled cell proliferation, hinder DNA repair mechanisms, and prevent the elimination of irreversibly mutated cells. Restrictive vegetarian and vegan diets may even increase the risk of vitamin and mineral deficiencies (especially vitamin B12, calcium, iron and zinc), haemorrhagic stroke (the rupture of a weakened blood vessel) and bone fractures.

Therefore, when transitioning to any diet, particularly restrictive ones like a vegan diet, whether practised full-time or a few days a week, it is crucial to understand what nutrients are essential for optimal health. In the following pages, we will outline the key components of a nutritious whole-foods, plant-based diet to ensure you gain all the health benefits while avoiding the pitfalls of unbalanced vegetarian diets.

The Longevity Diet: lessons from Blue Zones and historical contrasts

In regions known for high longevity, such as the Blue Zones, diets are predominantly plant-focused. These dietary patterns feature a rich array of colourful vegetables, minimally processed whole grains or sweet potatoes, beans, nuts, seeds and fish, with meat consumed sparingly. These diets are rich in fibre and essential nutrients while being low in empty calories, promoting improved health and longevity. On the other hand, historical evidence indicates that hunter – gatherer populations, such as indigenous groups in America, Australia, Africa, Mongolia and Greenland, who relied heavily on lean meat from wild game such as bison, kangaroo, boar, deer or seal, and had no access to refined or processed foods, seldom reached the age of 90.

The remarkable difference in longevity isn't merely due to modern medicine, as regions such as Okinawa and Sardinia, which had high numbers of healthy nonagenarians and centenarians long before the advent of contemporary medical advancements, demonstrate exceptional longevity rooted in their diet and lifestyle.

A growing body of scientific research on the biology of healthy aging supports these observations and underscores the crucial importance of a predominantly plant-based diet for promoting health and longevity, along with many other key lifestyle factors, which are summarised in the Healthy Longevity Code. Current evidence suggests that a meat-free diet is not strictly necessary to promote healthy aging and for preventing common chronic diseases such as cardiovascular disease, stroke, cancer, dementia and many inflammatory and autoimmune conditions. While the long-term benefits of consuming 'healthy' plant-centric diets appear substantial, it remains unclear whether less restrictive plant-rich diets, such as pescatarian or traditional Mediterranean-like diets, offer specific advantages regarding health outcomes like haemorrhagic stroke (a burst blood vessel in the brain that causes bleeding and brain cell damage) and bone fractures, which are sometimes associated with vegan diets. Further research is needed to better understand these effects and optimise dietary recommendations.

Nonetheless, if you decide to eliminate meat or all animal products for ethical, environmental, religious or philosophical reasons, it's crucial to recognise that not all plant foods are equally healthy. According to the American and Canadian dietetic associations, well-planned and properly supplemented vegan and lacto-ovo vegetarian diets can provide adequate nutrition throughout life and offer health benefits, including the prevention of some of the most common chronic diseases. However, as we have already discussed, vegetarian diets high in refined grains, hydrogenated oils, high-fructose corn syrup, sucrose, artificial sweeteners, salt and preservatives – typically found in ultra-processed foods, fast foods, and snacks – do not reduce mortality rates but instead increase the risk of disease and premature death.

These conclusions are supported by a robust body of evidence, including basic science, cross-sectional and prospective epidemiological studies, and an increasing number of randomised clinical trials, as outlined in our recent review published in the *European Heart Journal*,[1] the leading cardiovascular journal in the world. Vegetarian diets high in a balanced variety of minimally processed plant foods have been linked to a lower risk of developing various chronic diseases, including cardiovascular disease, diabetes, hypertension, cancer and dementia. Randomised clinical trials have further confirmed that vegetarian diets can help prevent diabetes, hypercholesterolemia, hypertension and obesity. However, there is currently no causal evidence from randomised trials on their impact on acute coronary syndrome, heart failure, stroke, cognitive impairment or dementia, and very limited data on cancer. Given the rising global adoption of vegetarian diets for ideological, cultural, environmental and personal reasons, it is crucial to identify which types of plant-based diets yield the best health outcomes and which components of vegetarian or vegan diets may be harmful.

1. Wang T, Masedunskas A, Willett WC, Fontana L. Vegetarian and vegan diets: benefits and drawbacks. Eur Heart J. 2023 Sep 21;44(36):3423-3439.

Key elements of a healthy plant-based diet

Recent advancements in our understanding of the metabolic and molecular mechanisms regulating aging have greatly improved our ability to make informed dietary and lifestyle choices that maximise health, wellbeing and longevity (see Figure 1). With this deeper knowledge, we can now more precisely determine what to eat, how much to consume, and when to engage in various activities to meet our nutritional, physical, emotional and spiritual needs.

Promoting health and longevity relies heavily on maintaining a healthy diet – arguably the most crucial factor, much like the king in a game of chess. Optimising diet quality while minimising 'empty' calories is essential for metabolic health. A primarily plant-based, fibre-rich diet, ideally supplemented with fish and low-fat dairy, serves as the foundation for improving both traditional and emerging risk factors through synergistic and complementary metabolic, molecular and metagenomic mechanisms.

Our diets should be carefully balanced to provide the right amount of energy, essential amino acids (the building blocks of proteins), fatty acids, and both soluble and insoluble fibres, while ensuring

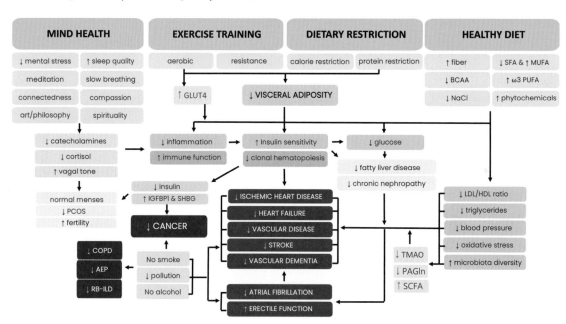

Figure 1 | Systems biology of healthy longevity and wellbeing

This figure illustrates the interconnected systems that promote health, wellbeing and longevity. By targeting common metabolic substrates, it is possible to proactively prevent a range of prevalent cardiometabolic and chronic diseases. Specific lifestyle interventions, which act through distinct yet complementary metabolic and molecular pathways, help prevent the accumulation of damage at the cellular, tissue and organ levels. Additionally, these interventions play a crucial role in modulating the development and progression of various chronic diseases, ultimately contributing to an extended health span. Abbreviations: PCOS, polycystic ovary syndrome; GLUT4, glucose transporter type 4; BCAA, branched-chain amino acids; NaCl, sodium chloride; SFA, saturated fatty acids; MUFA, monounsaturated fatty acids; PUFA, polyunsaturated fatty acids; IGFBP1, insulin-like growth factor binding protein-1; SHBG, sex hormone binding globulin; COPD, chronic obstructive pulmonary disease; AEP, acute eosinophilic pneumonia; RB-ILD, respiratory bronchiolitis-interstitial lung disease; LDL, low-density lipoprotein cholesterol; HDL, high-density lipoprotein cholesterol; TMAO, trimethylamine N-oxide; PAGln, phenylacetylglutamine; SCFA, short-chain fatty acids. Adapted from Cagigas ML, Twigg SM, Fontana L. Ten tips for promoting cardiometabolic health and slowing cardiovascular aging. Eur Heart J. 2024;45(13):1094-1097.

we meet 100 per cent of the recommended daily intake for every vitamin and mineral. Reducing the intake of saturated and trans fats, branched-chain and sulphur amino acids, and salt, while increasing the intake of fibre, polyunsaturated omega-3 fatty acids, essential vitamins (e.g., vitamins C, A, E, K, B complex, thiamine, niacin, biotin, folic acid and β-carotene), minerals (e.g., potassium, magnesium, phosphorus, manganese, selenium), and phytochemicals (e.g., polyphenols, terpenes, sterols and indoles), contributes significantly to these health benefits.

As illustrated in our food pyramid, vegetables form the foundation of any healthy diet, whether you are an omnivore or follow a plant-based regimen. Vegetables should make up the bulk of any diet. For many people, eating vegetables means consuming potatoes, tomatoes, lettuce, carrots and maybe some broccoli. Typically, this is what restaurants serve too. However, when we explore the diverse types of leaf, stem and root vegetables, we find that there are over 40 botanical families of vegetables, each offering hundreds of different varieties.

Examples of vegetables

Leafy greens: spinach, kale, lettuce, endive, collard greens, Swiss chard, dandelion greens, watercress, turnip greens, artichoke

Stalk vegetables: celery, asparagus, fennel, rhubarb, bamboo shoots

Root vegetables: carrot, beetroot, radish, turnip, potato, ginger, cassava

Cruciferous vegetables: broccoli, cauliflower, Brussels sprouts, cabbage, rocket (arugula)

Alliums: onion, garlic, leek, shallot, chives

Nightshades: tomato, capsicum, chilli, eggplant (aubergine)

Squash: zucchini (courgette), butternut squash, pumpkin, acorn squash

Gourds: cucumber, bitter melon

Mushrooms: button mushrooms, portobello, shiitake, oyster mushrooms

Findings from a randomised clinical trial of men and women without pre-existing cardiovascular disease show that consuming a diet rich in vegetables and fruits caused a significant reduction in markers of subclinical cardiac damage (high-sensitivity troponin I, N-terminal pro – B-type natriuretic peptide) in only eight weeks. A healthy primarily plant-centric fibre-rich diet also includes:

- minimally processed whole grains (e.g., brown rice, wheat, spelt, barley, millet, rye, corn, buckwheat)

- legumes (e.g., chickpeas, lentils, soy, black, kidney, pinto, navy, cannellini, adzuki and fava beans)

- nuts (walnuts, almonds, cashews, pistachios, hazelnuts, pecans, macadamia nuts, Brazil and pine nuts)

- seeds (flaxseeds, sesame, sunflower, pumpkin and chia seeds)

- low-glycaemic fruits (e.g., strawberries, raspberries, blackberries, blueberries, cherries, kiwifruit, plums, peaches, apples, pears, grapefruit, oranges)

- unsaturated fats (such as extra-virgin olive oil, avocados).

Depending on personal preferences, it may also incorporate moderate amounts of eggs, low-fat dairy and fish.

A diet that consistently incorporates these food groups at each meal provides a robust foundation for balanced nutrition, delivering essential vegetable fibres, complex carbohydrates, amino acids, vitamins, minerals, sterols, and polyphenols.

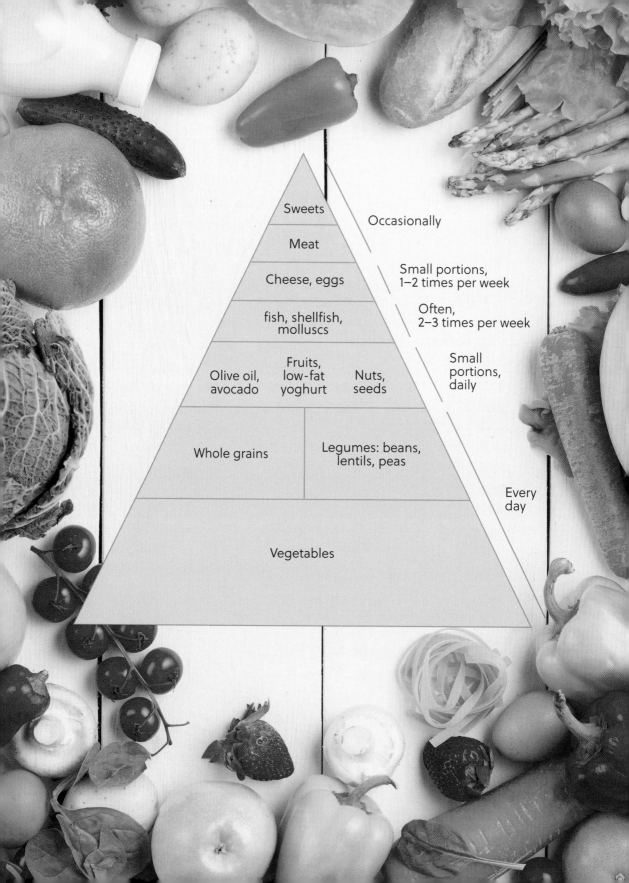

Sweets — Occasionally

Meat

Cheese, eggs — Small portions, 1–2 times per week

fish, shellfish, molluscs — Often, 2–3 times per week

Olive oil, avocado | Fruits, low-fat yoghurt | Nuts, seeds — Small portions, daily

Whole grains | Legumes: beans, lentils, peas

Vegetables — Every day

Over time, such a fibre- and water-rich diet can effectively lower LDL cholesterol (also called 'bad' cholesterol), glucose, insulin levels, inflammatory cytokines and blood pressure, while promoting a healthy weight. Additionally, it supports various metabolic pathways crucial for minimising cellular and tissue damage as you age (see Figure 1). Furthermore, by maintaining lower levels of choline, L-carnitine and phenylalanine – nutrients found in higher concentrations in red meat, eggs and cheese – this diet fosters a healthy gut microbiome. A well-balanced microbiome is vital for optimal immune function, as well as heart and brain health.

Eating minimally processed plant-based diets rich in fibre is key for weight loss

Regular endurance and resistance exercise is essential for maintaining or losing weight, but it's not sufficient on its own. Our research highlights the importance of a diet rich in vegetable fibre for effective calorie control, weight loss, and enhanced cardiometabolic health. In a randomised trial I conducted at Washington University in St. Louis, we replaced participants' typical diet of meat and highly processed food with minimally processed plant foods and fish, while keeping their caloric intake constant. Their meals included whole grains, beans, nuts, vegetables, low-fat yogurt, oat porridge and fish, while avoiding red meat, trans fats, refined carbs and sugar. With a daily fibre intake of 45 g – three times the average in Western diets – participants quickly began losing weight. To stabilise their weight and focus on the metabolic benefits of a high-quality diet, we added a daily surplus of 200 – 300 calories. This allowed us to assess the effects of the diet without the confounding factor of weight loss.

Natural fibre-rich foods such as vegetables, whole grains and legumes are key to promoting early satiety by increasing gastric distension, slowing gastric emptying and extending small bowel transit time. Fibre also stimulates the production of incretin hormones like GLP-1, which aids in weight loss, similar to the effects of the obesity drug *Ozempic®* (semaglutide), a once-weekly injectable GLP-1 receptor agonist. The lower energy density of plant-sourced foods also plays a crucial role in weight management. For instance, while you can quickly eat a large portion of white rice, a smaller serving of brown rice can provide the same level of satiety. Similarly, 100 g of Parmesan cheese contains around 384 calories, 28 g of fat and no fibre. In contrast, 100 g of cooked chickpeas has only 164 calories, 2.6 g of fat, 27 g of carbohydrates (including 7 g of fibre) and 9 g of protein. Whole-food vegan and vegetarian diets can result in fewer available calories to the body, leading to significant improvements in glucose tolerance, insulin sensitivity, blood pressure, and numerous cardiometabolic, inflammatory and hormonal factors linked to cardiovascular disease and cancer. In summary, to improve your health and manage your weight effectively over the long term, prioritise cutting out processed foods and significantly reducing animal products. Instead, focus on including more whole, natural plant-based foods in your diet.

The updated food pyramid

You probably first saw a food pyramid when you were at school. Not surprisingly, as our knowledge of health and wellbeing has evolved, so has the pyramid. These days, the base of the pyramid is made up of foods you should include in your diet every day, even at every meal. You should eat as many different varieties and colours of vegetables as you can, not just a few times a week, but most times you sit down at the table.

These should be accompanied by the next section of the pyramid: legumes and whole grains. All of these, as well as the nuts and seeds on the third tier of the pyramid, should be minimally processed.

The third tier also includes fruit. Many people exclude fruit from their diets due to its sugar and fructose content. Fruit rightly earns its place in the food pyramid due to its vitamins and minerals, which make fruit great for your skin and general health. Plus, the dietary fibre it provides forms a gel-like substance that improves gut health and leaves you feeling fuller for longer. Consider including fruit as dessert or a small snack during the day. A cup of blueberries or strawberries is packed with vitamin C; mango contains vitamins A, C and E; and an organic apple eaten with the skin on is packed with fibre and a flavonoid called quercetin, which may have anti-cancer properties.

The tiers above this are where you'll find fish and shellfish, cheese and eggs, and meat. Recommendations suggest you should only eat fish and shellfish two to three times a week, cheese and eggs once or twice a week, and if you desire meat or poultry only occasionally. Take this into consideration and it's easy to surmise that, for optimum health, most people should already be eating a plant-focused diet almost all the time. The tips and recipes in this book will help you make the transition to a plant-based diet or, if you already are a vegetarian or vegan, ensure you're creating meals that provide a full complement of nutrients.

Metabolic and molecular mechanisms behind the benefits of plant-based diets

While we don't yet fully understand all the ways in which primarily plant-centric fibre-rich diets

contribute to lowering the risk of type 2 diabetes, hypertension, heart disease, stroke, cancer, dementia and other prevalent health issues, many interrelated and overlapping factors have been hypothesised to play a role. The five most important mechanisms, which can mediate the pro-health and pro-longevity effects of healthy plant-based diets, are: (1) cholesterol lowering effect, (2) protection against oxidative stress, inflammation and the formation of blood clots, (3) modification of hormones and growth factors involved in the development of some of the most common cancers, (4) inhibition of pro-aging pathways by specific amino acid restriction, and (4) gut microbiota-mediated production of metabolites influencing the health of the immune system.

Cholesterol crusher: how plant-based diets keep your heart healthy

Several factors explain why vegetarians have significantly lower levels of cholesterol, and lower again if they consume minimally processed plant foods. Vegetarians do not consume meat, and vegans also avoid milk, butter and dairy. Butter, cream, cheese, beef, lamb and pork contain high levels of saturated fats and low amounts of monounsaturated or polyunsaturated fats. Even lean cuts of beef may contain up to 4.5 g of saturated fat for each 100 g serving. One cup of whole milk contains 4.5 g of saturated fat, and one tablespoon of butter contains 102 kcal and 7 g of saturated fat. In contrast, one tablespoon of olive oil contains 119 kcal and only 1.9 g of saturated fatty acids.

Studies have shown a strong relationship between saturated fat intake, plasma cholesterol levels and ischemic heart disease. Substituting 5 per cent of energy intake from saturated fatty acids with a similar quantity of energy from polyunsaturated fats (nuts, seeds), monounsaturated fats (olive oil, avocado) or carbohydrates from whole grains is associated with a 25 per cent, 15 per cent and 9 per cent lower risk of atherosclerotic coronary heart disease, respectively. However, replacing saturated fats with carbohydrates from refined sources (e.g., white bread and rice, pastries and baked goods, sweets and candies) substantially increases the risk of developing coronary heart disease. Data from randomised clinical trials have demonstrated a cause – effect relationship between replacing saturated fat with vegetable-based polyunsaturated fats from nuts and seeds, and a 30 per cent decrease in the risk of coronary heart disease. In a six-month randomised clinical trial, incorporating various cholesterol-lowering foods – including nuts, soy protein, viscous fibres from oats, barley, and psyllium, and plant sterol ester-enriched margarine – led to a notable 13 per cent reduction in plasma LDL cholesterol levels.

Legumes, seeds and nuts are rich sources of both soluble and insoluble fibres, each playing a crucial role in supporting cardiovascular health. Soluble fibre, which dissolves in water to form a gel-like substance, helps lower blood cholesterol levels. It achieves this by binding to cholesterol and bile acids in the small intestine, preventing their absorption into the bloodstream. This binding process facilitates the excretion of cholesterol through faeces, leading to reduced cholesterol levels in the blood. Data from randomised controlled studies reveal that high intake of water-soluble fibres, prevalent in beans and fruits, significantly lowers cholesterol levels. Specifically, each additional gram of water-soluble fibre consumed reduces plasma LDL cholesterol by approximately 1.12 mg/L.

Insoluble fibre, on the other hand, adds bulk to the stool, promoting regular bowel movements and supporting healthy digestion. It also serves as a substrate for the gut microbiota, enabling the production of key anti-inflammatory metabolites that contribute to overall immune health. Moreover, foods high in dietary fibre and with a low glycemic index can help lower insulin production and increase the levels of short-chain fatty acids. These short-chain fatty acids have been shown to inhibit cholesterol synthesis, further aiding in the reduction of blood cholesterol levels.

In addition to their fibre content, legumes, nuts and seeds contain plant sterols and stanols. These compounds have a chemical structure similar to cholesterol, which allows them to compete with cholesterol for absorption in the gut. By blocking the absorption of cholesterol, plant sterols and stanols help lower the overall cholesterol levels in the bloodstream. This mechanism contributes significantly to improved cardiovascular health and reduces the risk of heart disease. For example, studies have indicated that regular consumption of nuts can decrease the risk of coronary heart disease by up to 60 per cent.

Antioxidant armour: plant-based diets defend against stress and inflammation

A well-rounded plant-based diet – abundant in vegetables, fruits, legumes, minimally processed whole grains, nuts, seeds and extra-virgin olive oil – offers a rich array of antioxidants, including beta-carotene, vitamins C and E, natural folate, flavonoids and selenium. For instance, a thoughtfully crafted vegetarian diet can provide approximately 6000 µg of beta-carotene, 17 mg of vitamin E, 400 µg of natural folate, 300 mg of flavonoids and 120 µg of selenium daily.

Oxidative stress is a major contributor to chronic conditions such as heart disease, cancer and dementia. A landmark international study known as INTER-HEART, which involved over 27,000 participants across 52 countries, found that dietary antioxidants might help protect against heart disease. A low intake of antioxidants from vegetables is associated with a higher risk of atherosclerosis, a condition where plaque builds up in the arteries due to the oxidation of lipoproteins. Lipoproteins are tiny particles in your blood that transport fats, such as cholesterol and triglycerides, throughout your body. Among these, low-density lipoproteins (LDL) are often referred to as 'bad' cholesterol because they can contribute to plaque formation in the arteries. Elevated levels of oxidised LDL are an independent marker of atherosclerosis and heart disease. Recent clinical trials suggest that a Mediterranean-style diet, rich in whole plant foods, nuts and extra-virgin olive oil, can significantly lower levels of oxidised LDL and inflammation markers. Since oxidative and inflammatory damage are closely intertwined, they both contribute to the early stages of atherosclerosis.

While the specific foods or nutrients responsible for the anti-inflammatory benefits of a plant-based diet are not yet fully understood, it is believed that the combined effects of various nutrients from a range of plant foods play a significant role. This may be due to interactions with gut microbiota and improvements in gut health, such as reduced permeability, which collectively help lower inflammation. Research indicates that individuals who consume higher-quality plant-centric diets tend to have lower inflammation levels, even when traditional risk factors are considered. On the other hand, some foods can independently increase inflammation. For example, trans fats are associated with increased inflammation, endothelial dysfunction (impaired blood vessel lining that affects blood pressure and clotting) and a higher risk of type 2 diabetes. In contrast, omega-3 fatty acids are linked to reduced inflammation and lower triglyceride levels. Omega-3s help decrease inflammation by interacting

with a specific receptor in the body, known as G-protein – coupled receptor 120, and by inhibiting the activity of a protein complex called the NLRP3 inflammasome, which triggers inflammation.

Whole grains, legumes and extra-virgin olive oil contain several phytochemicals that contribute to their anti-inflammatory and antioxidant properties. For example, the aleurone layer of wheat bran is rich in compounds such as ferulic acid, alkylresorcinols, apigenin, lignans and phytic acid, which have been shown to possess antioxidant and anti-inflammatory effects and may help protect against cancer in preclinical studies. Wholemeal flour, which has a total phenolic acid content ranging from 71 to 87 mg/g, contains over 80 per cent of this as ferulic acid. Additionally, the germ of whole grains contains spermidine, a polyamine that has been found to extend lifespan in various experimental organisms and human cells by reducing oxidative stress, boosting autophagy and lowering inflammation.

Cold-pressed extra-virgin olive oil is a rich source of antioxidants. A 100 g serving (about seven tablespoons) contains up to 25 mg of α-tocopherol (vitamin E) and 1 – 2 mg of carotenoids, both of which are effective antioxidants. It also provides 20 – 500 mg of oleuropein and 98 – 185 mg of phytosterols. Freshly pressed extra-virgin olive oil contains up to 9 mg of oleocanthal, a compound that imparts a pungent sensation and has anti-inflammatory properties similar to ibuprofen. Although this amount may not have a strong anti-inflammatory effect on its own, it can still help protect against platelet aggregation and coronary thrombosis, much like a low-dose aspirin.

Hormone harmony: plant-based eating and cancer prevention

Calorie restriction, without malnutrition, has been shown to be the most effective intervention to prevent cancer in animals and significantly reduces metabolic and hormonal factors linked to cancer and aging in humans. While a 'healthy' plant-based diet doesn't require strict calorie counting, studies show that replacing refined and processed (high-glycemic index) foods typical of the Western diet with minimally processed plant foods can lead to significant weight loss. For instance, in one study, women randomised to a primarily plant-rich diet lost almost 4 kg in only 5 months, and experienced a substantial reduction in fasting glucose, insulin and testosterone levels, along with increases in proteins that reduce the biological activity of insulin-like growth factor 1 (IGF-1), testosterone and estradiol.

Insulin, estrogens, androgens and IGF-1 are potent stimulators of cell growth and play a significant role in the development and progression of several common cancers, including breast, colon, prostate, pancreatic and endometrial cancers. It remains unclear whether these hormonal changes are primarily driven by diet quality, weight loss, or both. However, the reduction in body fat associated with a low-energy, high-fibre, plant-centric diet appears to be the main factor improving insulin sensitivity. This is supported by findings that the beneficial effects on insulin levels were no longer statistically significant after accounting for changes in weight and waist circumference.

While weight loss seems to be the primary driver, other aspects of plant-focused eating, such as its low glycemic index, high intake of monounsaturated and omega-3 fatty acids, and lower intake of branched-chain amino acids, may also contribute to reducing insulin resistance and compensatory hyperinsulinemia, which can accelerate aging and cancer development. Additionally, a diet high in fibre has been shown to increase faecal mass and enhance the excretion of estrogens, resulting in lower plasma levels of estrone and estradiol. This reduction in estrogen may help protect against hormone-related cancers, such as breast and ovarian cancer, by decreasing the levels of these growth-promoting hormones in the body. Moreover, a high-fibre diet offers direct protection against colon cancer, which is the second most common cancer in Western countries. Fibre contributes to this protective effect in several ways: it speeds up colonic transit time, which helps prevent the prolonged contact of carcinogenic substances with the intestinal lining. Additionally, fibre binds to these harmful substances, facilitating their removal from the digestive tract and reducing their absorption. This combined action not only lowers the risk of colon cancer but also supports overall digestive health and helps maintain a healthy gut microbiome, which can further contribute to cancer prevention and general health.

Finally, a healthy vegetarian diet is abundant in plant foods that contain compounds with potential protective effects against cancer. These beneficial compounds include:

- **Isothiocyanates, indol-3-carbinol and sulforaphane:** Found in cruciferous vegetables like broccoli, cabbage and Brussels sprouts, these compounds are known for their ability to detoxify carcinogens and inhibit cancer cell growth.

- **Organosulfur compounds:** Found in onions and garlic, these compounds have been shown to inhibit cancer cell proliferation, metastasis and cell cycle progression. They do this by activating several metabolising enzymes, such as cytochrome P450s, which help to activate or detoxify carcinogens, and glutathione S-transferases, which aid in their detoxification. Additionally, organosulfur compounds can prevent the formation of DNA adducts in various tissues, thereby reducing cancer risk.

This vegetarian life

Anuja, 29, has been pescatarian for two years.

'I'm vegetarian most days of the week, but also eat fish and seafood occasionally – usually when I'm eating out or travelling.

'I've tried to go vegetarian a few times in the past, but now I've been off meat for two years. Every now and then, if there's a delicious goat curry, I'll have the gravy, but I don't crave meat or need it to feel full anymore.

'Initially I cut meat from my diet for health reasons, out of curiosity to see how I would feel and whether I would have more energy. The first few weeks were difficult because I never felt full, so I would load up on carbs, which made me feel lethargic. But I stuck with it for a few months and it got easier. I lost weight, my stomach felt lighter, but I also developed low iron levels.

'I do feel like it's improved my health. The most tangible difference is in my energy levels. I don't have as many crashes around midday as I used to have when I was eating meat for lunch or dinner. It helps me sleep better too since I don't feel like I'm going to bed on a heavy stomach. Plus, I get fewer upset stomachs compared to when I was eating meat.

'I've had to incorporate fish and seafood back into my meals due to my iron levels dropping and I also take B12 supplements. But I've since found workarounds like eating more lentils during the week, which is great since I love dahl and lentil soups!

'Another reason I've incorporated seafood is because, although I'm not vegan, I'm lactose intolerant. If I'm eating out, seafood and fish usually don't have dairy, so again, it's a way to eat something that's actually tasty.

'I think my heritage, being Indian, has made it a lot easier for me to maintain a vegetarian diet since a significant portion of the food I grew up with was vegetarian.'

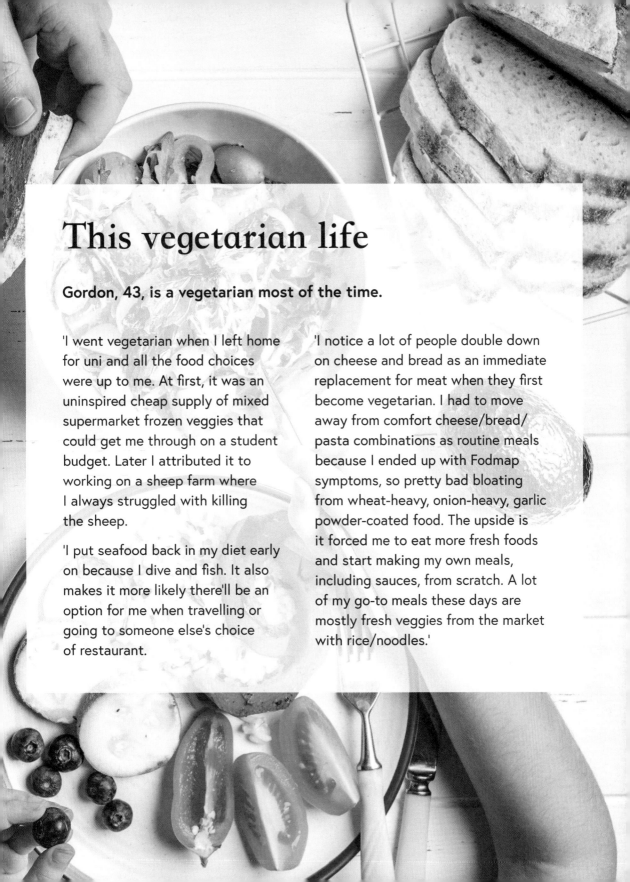

This vegetarian life

Gordon, 43, is a vegetarian most of the time.

'I went vegetarian when I left home for uni and all the food choices were up to me. At first, it was an uninspired cheap supply of mixed supermarket frozen veggies that could get me through on a student budget. Later I attributed it to working on a sheep farm where I always struggled with killing the sheep.

'I put seafood back in my diet early on because I dive and fish. It also makes it more likely there'll be an option for me when travelling or going to someone else's choice of restaurant.

'I notice a lot of people double down on cheese and bread as an immediate replacement for meat when they first become vegetarian. I had to move away from comfort cheese/bread/ pasta combinations as routine meals because I ended up with Fodmap symptoms, so pretty bad bloating from wheat-heavy, onion-heavy, garlic powder-coated food. The upside is it forced me to eat more fresh foods and start making my own meals, including sauces, from scratch. A lot of my go-to meals these days are mostly fresh veggies from the market with rice/noodles.'

- **Lycopene:** A powerful antioxidant found in tomatoes, lycopene is associated with a reduced risk of prostate cancer and other cancers due to its ability to neutralise free radicals and prevent the oxidative damage of DNA.

- **Polyacetylenes:** Present in vegetables such as carrots, celery and parsley, these compounds demonstrate strong cytotoxic effects against various cancer cells. They also help to reduce inflammation and oxidative stress, contributing to their cancer-fighting properties.

- **Monoterpenes** (carvacrol and linalool): Found in citrus fruits like oranges and lemons, inhibit tumour growth in both laboratory and animal studies. They work through various mechanisms, including triggering programmed cell death of mutated cells (apoptosis), disrupting the cell cycle, and promoting processes like autophagy and necroptosis, which help combat cancer.

- **Capsaicin:** The active compound in chillis, capsaicin alters the expression of several genes that arrest the cell cycle in tumour cells and promotes apoptosis.

- **Quercitin and Ginkgetin:** Found in capers, this compound has demonstrated potential anti-cancer effects by inhibiting cancer cell proliferation by controlling the activity of oncogenic and tumour suppressor genes such as ncRNAs.

- **Ferulic acid and spermidine:** Found in whole grains, these compounds have antioxidant, anti-inflammatory and autophagic properties that contribute to their cancer-protective effects.

Among these, specific phytoestrogens such as formononetin, biochanin A, coumestans, genistein, and daidzein – particularly abundant in beans, especially fava beans and lupin – play a crucial role. These low-potency estrogenic molecules can compete with endogenous estrogens for binding to estrogen receptors. By doing so, they can block the mitogenic effects of stronger natural estrogens, potentially reducing the risk of estrogen-related cancers such as breast and ovarian cancer. This competitive binding helps to modulate estrogen activity in the body, offering another layer of protection against hormone-driven cancer development.

Aging defence: the power of amino acid restriction in plant-based diets

A whole-food, plant-centric diet generally provides about 20 per cent less protein compared to a typical Western diet. In practice, this means that a healthy vegetarian diet usually contains around 70 g of protein per day, while a Western diet, which is often high in animal products, typically includes at least 90 g of protein. In a plant-based diet, most of the protein is sourced from plant-based foods such as legumes, whole grains and nuts. For instance, people following a plant-heavy diet consume an average of at least 40 g of protein from whole grains and legumes alone. Additionally, nuts and seeds contribute to overall protein intake.

Why is this important? Recent preclinical studies show that moderate reduction in protein intake can extend lifespan, regardless of the total calorie intake. In various animal models, including rodents, cutting back on protein or swapping animal proteins for plant proteins has been shown to inhibit the growth of prostate and breast cancer, leading to a reduced activity of a key pathway involved in aging and cancer, known as mTOR. Consistently, a recent epidemiological study found that individuals aged 50 – 65 who consumed the most protein (more than 20 per cent of their daily calories) had a 75 per cent higher overall mortality rate and were four times more likely to die from cancer. However, these risks were either reduced or eliminated when the protein came from plant-based sources. Additionally, several studies suggest that a high-protein diet is linked to an increased risk of obesity, cardiovascular disease and type 2 diabetes. For instance, the risk of developing type 2 diabetes rises by 20 – 40 per cent for every 10 g of protein consumed above 64 g per day.

In a well-designed clinical trial, the use of whey protein supplements in a calorie-restricted weight-loss diet did not result in the expected improvements in insulin sensitivity that are typically seen with a 10 per cent weight loss in women with obesity. This suggests that whey protein supplementation might interfere with the metabolic benefits usually associated with weight loss. In contrast, another randomised clinical trial observed different outcomes. Overweight and mildly obese middle-aged men who followed a moderately protein-restricted diet for 4 – 6 weeks experienced notable health improvements. This diet led to significant reductions in body weight and fat mass, as well as decreases in fasting blood glucose levels and C-reactive protein, a marker of inflammation. Additionally, these men saw a substantial increase in circulating levels of FGF21, a hormone linked to enhanced metabolic health and increased longevity.

Beyond just the amount of protein, the type of protein may also be more important. The vegetarian diet's markedly lower intake of animal protein means it has different levels of essential amino acids compared to a Western diet. For instance, the intake of methionine, an essential amino acid, is about 40 per cent lower in a healthy plant-based diet. This is significant because methionine restriction in experimental animal models has consistently been shown to extend lifespan and protect against chronic diseases, particularly cancer. In rodents, reducing methionine improves glucose metabolism, protects against obesity and fatty liver, and lowers oxidative stress. Methionine restriction also triggers changes in hormone levels similar to those seen in animals on a calorie-restricted diet, which is known to promote longevity.

Other essential amino acids like leucine, isoleucine, valine and tryptophan are also consumed at lower levels in vegetarian diets compared to the Western diet. Research indicates that these branched-chain amino acids (BCAAs) are important in regulating insulin sensitivity. Elevated levels of BCAAs are found in people and animals with insulin resistance, and high consumption of these amino acids has been linked to an 11 – 13 per cent increased risk of developing type 2 diabetes. Moreover, a recent study in rodents showed that selectively reducing the intake of BCAAs significantly improved glucose tolerance, reduced stress on insulin-producing cells, and improved body composition.

At the cellular level, our bodies detect essential amino acids through specific nutrient-sensing pathways, with two key ones being mTOR and GCN2. The mTOR pathway, which is linked to aging and cancer, gets activated by calorie intake and a cocktail of different essential amino acids, especially methionine, leucine and isoleucine. On the other hand, when specific amino acids are limited, the GCN2 pathway kicks in, triggering a protective response in cells. In simple terms, eating a plant-centric high-fibre diet, which typically has lower protein content, especially from animal sources, might be a key factor in its health benefits. The type and quality of protein we consume, along with the balance of essential amino acids, can influence aging, disease risk, and overall health.

Gut health boost: how plant-based foods transform your microbiota

The trillions of microorganisms residing in our gut, collectively known as the gut microbiota, are essential to our overall health. These microorganisms produce a range of metabolites that impact our immune system, metabolism and inflammation levels. As highlighted in one of our highly cited publications in the prestigious journal *Science*, diet – particularly the amounts of protein and fibre – plays a crucial role in determining the composition and function of these gut microbes. A healthy plant-based diet, for example, differs greatly from the typical Western diet, which is rich in choline and L-carnitine – nutrients found in high concentrations in red meat, eggs and cheese. Gut bacteria convert these substances into trimethylamine N-oxide (TMAO), a metabolite linked to a 20 per cent increased risk of cardiovascular diseases like heart attacks and strokes. TMAO can also cause blood vessel inflammation and increase blood clotting, with growing evidence suggesting it may contribute to obesity and type 2 diabetes. Additionally, higher levels of phenylacetylglutamine, a metabolite produced from the gut's processing of the amino acid phenylalanine – especially when consumed in excess – are associated with a dose-dependent increase in coronary heart disease risk. This risk is particularly elevated in women who consume more animal-based foods and fewer vegetable-based foods.

A stand-out feature of a healthy vegetarian diet rich in complex carbohydrates is its high fibre content, particularly insoluble fibre, which is more than double what's found in a typical Western diet. This fibre feeds beneficial gut bacteria, leading to an increase in helpful species like Bacteroidetes, which produce short-chain fatty acids (SCFAs) such as acetate, propionate and butyrate. These SCFAs are known to have anti-inflammatory and immune-modulating effects and may help prevent diseases like allergies and autoimmune disorders. Some of these benefits are thought to occur because SCFAs can activate specific receptors on immune cells and cells lining the gut. In a recent study, obese individuals who followed a plant-based Mediterranean-like diet for two years experienced significant changes in their gut bacteria. There was a rise in beneficial bacteria like Bacteroides, Prevotella, Faecalibacterium, and especially Roseburia and Ruminococcus. These bacteria are experts at breaking down carbohydrates into SCFAs. Notably, certain species like Faecalibacterium prausnitzii and Bacteroides fragilis were shown to promote the production of an anti-inflammatory molecule called interleukin-10. Another study found that people who closely followed a plant-centric Mediterranean diet had more beneficial gut bacteria and higher levels of SCFAs in their stool. Conversely, those with poor adherence to the diet had higher levels of harmful bacteria and a rise in TMAO levels.

It appears that sticking to a healthy plant-focused dietary pattern over the long term has a more significant and lasting effect on gut bacteria than short-term dietary changes. As demonstrated in our scientific article published in *Cell Host & Microbe*, a diet rich in plant-based foods and low in calories is associated with a more diverse and healthier gut microbiota. Conversely, adhering to a Western-like diet over multiple generations, which often lacks essential nutrients for gut bacteria, can lead to a decline in certain beneficial bacterial species. This reduction in microbial diversity may impair immune function and elevate the risk of developing various metabolic, inflammatory and autoimmune diseases.

Unhealthy vegetarian diets

Refined carbs, sweets and
sugar-sweetened beverages
Vegetarian ultra-processed foods
Trans-fats and tropical oils

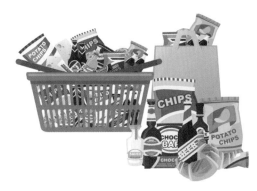

Healthy vegetarian diets

Vegetables, fruits and nuts
Whole grains, legumes, nuts, seeds
Unsaturated fats
Low-fat dairy and eggs

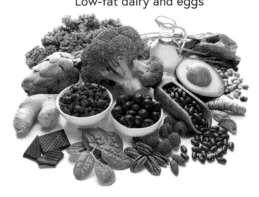

Put quality on the table

Understanding how a balanced plant-focused diet supports metabolic and molecular health is essential, but equally important is grasping the fundamentals of culinary science to enhance overall wellbeing. Knowing the specific characteristics of different food groups, including their nutrient profiles and the optimal methods for pairing and preparing them, is crucial for maximising their health benefits. The quality of the ingredients we choose for cooking has a profound impact on our health. Selecting fresh, nutrient-dense foods and employing proper cooking techniques not only preserves and enhances their nutritional value but also influences their taste and texture. For example, lightly steaming vegetables can help retain more vitamins compared to boiling them, while incorporating a variety of herbs and spices can boost flavour without added sodium. Furthermore, the sources of our ingredients and the methods used to prepare them reflect broader practices in agriculture and culinary arts. Sustainable farming practices and environmentally friendly food preparation techniques contribute to both personal health and the health of our planet. Choosing locally sourced, organic produce and reducing food waste are examples of how culinary choices can align with environmental sustainability goals.

To make this concept clearer, think of food as similar to the colours used by a master painter. Just as the quality of the pigments and their blending with the medium, like linseed oil, is crucial for creating a stunning and long-lasting painting, the quality of the foods we use is vital for crafting nutritious and flavourful meals. In painting, the effectiveness of the colours depends on their purity, intensity, and resistance to fading. Similarly, the nutritional value and taste of our meals are significantly influenced by the quality of the ingredients. Premium paints lead to a more vibrant and enduring artwork, just as high-quality

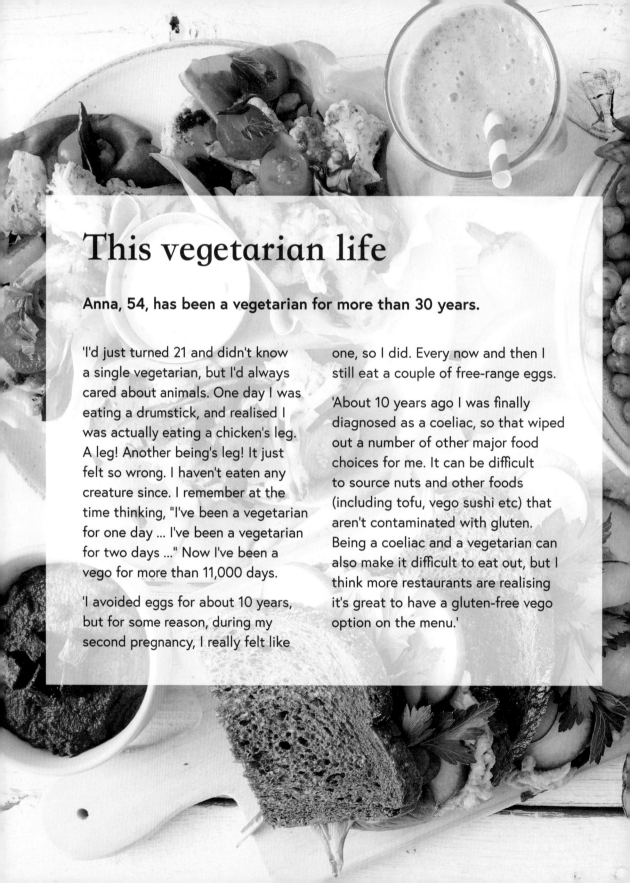

This vegetarian life

Anna, 54, has been a vegetarian for more than 30 years.

'I'd just turned 21 and didn't know a single vegetarian, but I'd always cared about animals. One day I was eating a drumstick, and realised I was actually eating a chicken's leg. A leg! Another being's leg! It just felt so wrong. I haven't eaten any creature since. I remember at the time thinking, "I've been a vegetarian for one day ... I've been a vegetarian for two days ..." Now I've been a vego for more than 11,000 days.

'I avoided eggs for about 10 years, but for some reason, during my second pregnancy, I really felt like one, so I did. Every now and then I still eat a couple of free-range eggs.

'About 10 years ago I was finally diagnosed as a coeliac, so that wiped out a number of other major food choices for me. It can be difficult to source nuts and other foods (including tofu, vego sushi etc) that aren't contaminated with gluten. Being a coeliac and a vegetarian can also make it difficult to eat out, but I think more restaurants are realising it's great to have a gluten-free vego option on the menu.'

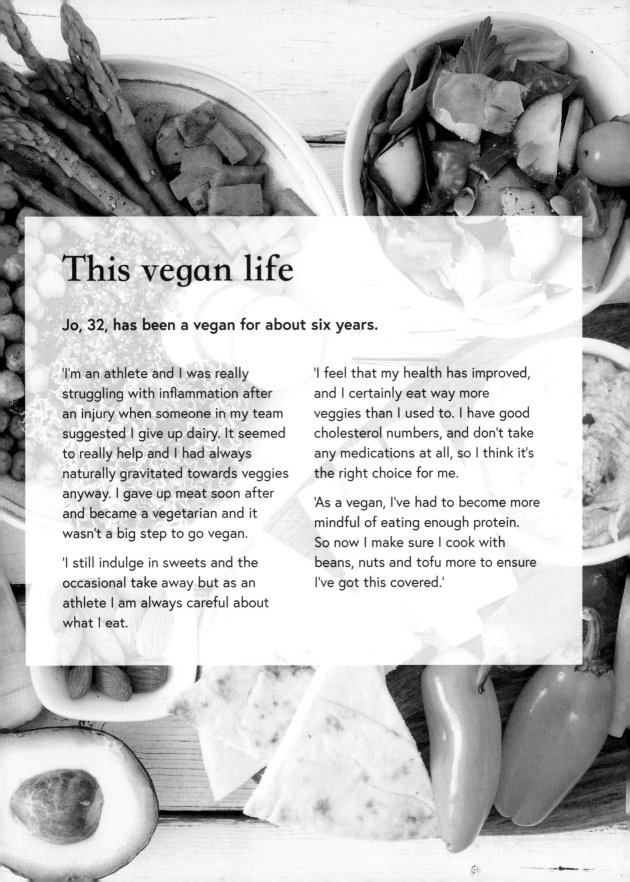

This vegan life

Jo, 32, has been a vegan for about six years.

'I'm an athlete and I was really struggling with inflammation after an injury when someone in my team suggested I give up dairy. It seemed to really help and I had always naturally gravitated towards veggies anyway. I gave up meat soon after and became a vegetarian and it wasn't a big step to go vegan.

'I still indulge in sweets and the occasional take away but as an athlete I am always careful about what I eat.

'I feel that my health has improved, and I certainly eat way more veggies than I used to. I have good cholesterol numbers, and don't take any medications at all, so I think it's the right choice for me.

'As a vegan, I've had to become more mindful of eating enough protein. So now I make sure I cook with beans, nuts and tofu more to ensure I've got this covered.'

ingredients contribute to a healthier and more enjoyable dining experience. Choosing ingredients with care is akin to selecting the finest pigments for a masterpiece. Ingredients that are sustainably sourced and thoughtfully prepared off er enhanced health benefits, richer flavours, and better overall nutrition. They contribute to both physical wellbeing and emotional satisfaction, much like how exceptional colours and techniques result in a remarkable painting.

Eating well to stay healthy is all about quality and variety. This isn't just a good idea; it's a fundamental principle of nature. For example, monocultures in agriculture often lead to problems like diseases and pests, which then need to be controlled with pesticides and herbicides. Nature thrives on diversity. Similarly, our diets should be as diverse as possible. This doesn't mean 'a little bit of everything', including unhealthy foods, but rather following the best scientific advice and learning from the dietary habits of populations known for their health and longevity. The Mediterranean diet and the diet of the centenarians from Okinawa are excellent examples of this. Their diets, as we have already discussed, are rich in a wide variety of minimally processed foods, mainly plant-powered but not exclusively so. This diversity is a key factor in their protective, health-promoting eff ects, helping the people in these regions live longer and healthier lives, while avoiding malnutrition.

Therefore, to ensure you're eating healthy and at the same time meeting your nutritional needs, focus on removing refined and processed food and beverages from your diet and replace them with minimally processed plant-based foods that that are rich in nutrients and low in harmful elements. Even if you choose to eat meat occasionally, the bulk of your meals should consist of vegetables, legumes, nuts, seeds, fruit and whole grains. Incorporating a wide diversity of each to ensure you're receiving the broad range of the nutrients, vitamins, antioxidants, oligoelements, phytochemicals and soluble/insoluble fibres your body needs for maximum health.

If you've chosen to practise vegetarianism, whether at every meal or just some of them, to improve your health, fill your fridge and cupboards with the freshest and most nutritionally dense food you can find. Evidence suggests that some vegetarians, especially those following more restrictive diets like veganism, may be at higher risk for deficiencies in essential nutrients such as vitamin B12, riboflavin, iron, zinc, calcium and omega-3 fatty acids if they do not carefully plan their diets and include fortified plant-based foods or supplements. This risk is particularly significant for pregnant and breastfeeding women, as well as growing children, who require these nutrients for proper development. To ensure that a restrictive vegetarian or vegan diet is nutritionally balanced, it is advisable for individuals to consult with a registered dietitian or healthcare provider.

If you decide to include red meat and poultry in your diet, it's important to consider not only their potential chronic health impacts but also the quality of the products you consume. Unfortunately, about two-thirds of animals raised for food in most industrialised countries are kept in factory farms, where they are often treated as mere commodities. These industrial operations focus on maximising production and minimising costs, often at the expense of animal welfare, subjecting billions of animals to overcrowded, unsanitary and stressful conditions. In these factory farms, animals are deprived of basic freedoms like sunlight, fresh air and a natural diet. Many chickens, for instance, spend their entire lives crammed into tiny wire cages that severely restrict movement. Calves and pigs are confined to cramped metal stalls or windowless sheds, preventing them from engaging in natural behaviours such as caring for their young, building nests, or foraging. Dairy cows endure particularly harsh treatment, including the removal of their horn buds early in life and repeated cycles of artificial insemination to keep them producing milk. When their milk production declines, they are sent to slaughter. Similarly, young steers are quickly processed into hamburger meat after minimal time in feedlots. These inhumane conditions, coupled with poor-quality feed and the excessive use of antibiotics and sometimes hormones, adversely affect the quality of the meat, milk and eggs that end up on your plates. The realities of factory farming are often hidden from consumers, but awareness of how these animals are treated can lead to a reassessment of regular consumption of these products.

Harmony on your plate: blending pleasure and health in plant-centric eating

Pleasure and health should not be viewed as conflicting goals to be wrestled with daily. Instead, they can be harmonised to enrich both our lives and our dining experiences. A well-crafted dish is much more than just food: it's a culinary masterpiece. The quality of the ingredients, the techniques used in their preparation, their textures, flavours, aromas and colours, along with the creative balance achieved, all blend to create a symphony of sensory delight that dances upon our tastebuds, enchants our eyes, tantalises our sense of smell and awakens our palate with its textural sensations, while uplifting our soul.

In the following sections of this book, we will explore how the art of selecting, combining, transforming, and savouring food can become a mindful practice that enhances creativity and

emotional wellbeing. To fully appreciate and be inspired by the culinary expertise of our chef-in-residence, Marzio Lanzini, it's essential to gain a deep understanding of the ingredients used. While we will use traditional food categories for clarity, it is crucial to remember – something we will emphasise throughout this chapter – that fats, proteins and carbohydrates should not be viewed as generic categories. Each food item must be evaluated on its individual qualities. For example, there is a notable difference between a loaf of bread made from highly processed white flour and one made from freshly milled wholegrain flour and natural sourdough. These distinctions significantly impact both health and enjoyment, despite both being classified as carbohydrates.

We hope this book will inspire readers to move beyond simplistic food classifications and embrace a more nuanced understanding of nutrition. Ultimately, this chapter aims to reinforce foundational concepts while guiding you to become more mindful consumers, creative architects of your diet, and responsible stewards of the planet. By adopting a more comprehensive view of food, you can enhance your health, elevate your culinary experiences and contribute to a more sustainable future.

Vegetables: your best dietary friend

There's a Latin word, *vegetabilis*, that means growing or flourishing. It's where the English word 'vegetable' comes from, and it's an apt derivation since vegetables are essential for flourishing health. A healthy and balanced diet must include a wide variety of these ingredients in abundance. It has been shown that they not only meet basic nutritional needs, but also provide many other beneficial substances for our health, such as the so-called phytochemicals, which are bioactive compounds. Scientific studies suggest that, when consumed in the right proportions, these molecules have antioxidant, anti-inflammatory, anti-cancer and immune-boosting properties. Therefore, they are essential in a balanced diet that helps us live well and longer.

They make up the base of the new food pyramid, with whole grains and legumes just above them, so these three types of food should make up the bulk of every meal you eat, whether you are a full-time vegetarian or only eat meat-free meals a couple of days a week.

Leafy green, orange-yellow and purple vegetables have the lowest caloric density but the highest concentration of healthy vitamins, minerals and oligoelements (trace elements). If you're trying to lose weight, the high fibre and water content of these veggies can be helpful. Research has proven the higher the intake of vegetables, the better the reduction in body weight and the healthier the gut microbiome.

Incorporating a diverse array of vegetables into your diet, especially when prepared with care, is instrumental in preventing a range of chronic diseases. Extensive research consistently demonstrates that diets rich in vegetables are linked to significantly reduced mortality rates. This reduction is particularly notable in cases of cardiovascular disease, various cancers, respiratory illnesses (including those linked to tobacco use) and digestive disorders.

Vegetables offer more than just essential nutrients; they also play a key role in maintaining an alkaline environment within the body. This is particularly important when consuming acidifying foods like meat, fish, and dairy products. By helping to balance the body's pH levels, vegetables support the delicate acid-base equilibrium that is crucial for the optimal functioning of our cells. This balance is fundamental to overall health, as it underpins vital processes such as cellular repair, immune system efficiency, energy production, and detoxification.

Vegetables are not only a boon for metabolic health – being the one food group with virtually no significant contraindications – but they also serve as an almost inexhaustible source of flavour, colour and creativity in the kitchen. The vast variety of vegetables can be categorised into leafy greens (lettuce, radicchio, endive, chicory, spinach, kale, chard, parsley, coriander, watercress, rocket, dandelion), flowering vegetables (artichoke, cauliflower, broccoli, asparagus, cardoon), fruiting vegetables (cucumber, zucchini, pumpkin, capsicum, eggplant, tomato, capers, olives), root vegetables (radish, carrot, beet, turnip), bulb vegetables (onion, garlic, shallot, leek, fennel) and an endless array of wild herbs. Each category offers a rich diversity of local ecotypes, where nutritional profiles and flavours are uniquely enhanced or subdued.

While many of us tend to stick to familiar vegetables like potatoes, carrots, peas and tomatoes, there is a world of other options waiting to be explored. Don't hesitate to experiment with new varieties, as each comes with its own distinct flavours and nutritional benefits. Whether sourced from your local greengrocer, farmers' market or your own garden, incorporating a diverse range of vegetables into your meals will provide a significant nutritional boost. Whenever possible, choose organic options to maximise health benefits and flavour.

It's a good idea to greatly reduce the number of white potatoes you consume. Research has shown eating them daily can put someone at a higher risk of developing type 2 diabetes. Eat them once a week, if you must, but never fried.

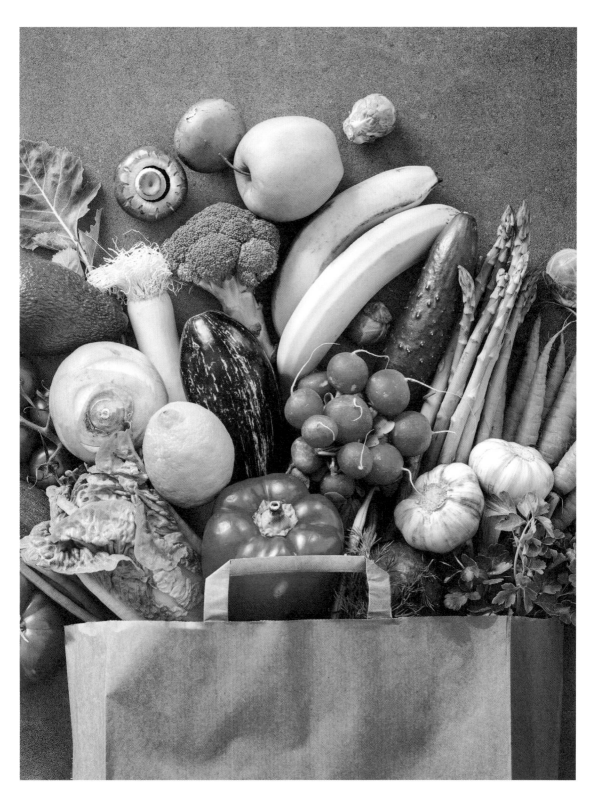

Protein plus

Protein, composed of amino acids, is the building block of life and an essential component of a healthy diet. The body relies on essential and non-essential amino acids to construct cellular organelles, tissues and organs. They are crucial for producing hormones and enzymes, as well as for building and repairing muscles and bones. A common misconception is that only animal products – such as meat, poultry, eggs and dairy – are rich sources of protein. However, this is not true. Plant-sourced foods also contain all the essential amino acids, albeit in varying proportions.

For example, legumes are rich in lysine but lower in tryptophan and methionine, while whole grains are low in lysine but high in tryptophan and methionine. When combined, such as in a meal of brown rice and lentils or durum wheat pasta with chickpeas, these plant foods provide a complete protein profile – equivalent to the protein found in eggs or meat. This is why it's important to combine whole grains and legumes, sometimes multiple times throughout the day, especially for those following a vegetarian or vegan diet.

Lentils, for instance, are not only budget-friendly and quick to prepare but also pack a significant protein punch. About a third of their calories come from protein, making them one of the highest-protein legumes by weight. Tempeh and tofu, both derived from soybeans, are also excellent sources of complete protein and are often considered nutritional powerhouses. A 100 g serving of tofu or tempeh provides 8 g of protein, along with carbohydrates, fibre and essential minerals such as manganese, calcium, selenium, phosphorus, copper, magnesium, iron and zinc, all for just 70 calories per serving.

In addition to these, incorporating nuts and seeds such as peanuts, almonds, pumpkin seeds, sunflower seeds, cashews and pistachios into your diet can further boost your protein intake. These plant options offer a generous amount of protein and other vital nutrients, making them a valuable addition to any diet. A meta-analysis of 31 prospective cohort studies suggests that intake of plant, but not animal protein, is associated with an 8 per cent lower risk of all-cause mortality, and 12 per cent lower cardiovascular disease mortality. For any additional 3 per cent increase in daily energy intake from plant proteins there was a linear 5 per cent lower all-causes mortality risk.

According to the 2021 American Heart Association guidelines, it's recommended to prioritise plant proteins, such as legumes, nuts and whole grains, for a heart-healthy diet. Fish and seafood are also advised, as they are rich sources of vitamin B12 and zinc. The guidelines suggest opting for low-fat or fat-free dairy products over full-fat versions to lower saturated fat intake and reduce levels of bad cholesterol in the blood. Importantly, for the first time, the guidelines emphasise that meat and poultry are not recommended but, if consumed, should be limited to lean cuts and strictly avoided in processed forms. This shift underscores a strong preference for plant-based options while acknowledging that meat should be considered only if absolutely desired. This represents a notable change towards dietary choices that enhance cardiometabolic health, support environmental sustainability, and minimise the risks associated with frequent consumption of both unprocessed and processed meats.

Beans and grains: the other benefits

While legumes (chickpeas, lentils, soy, black, kidney, pinto, navy, cannellini, adzuki and fava beans) and whole grains play an important role in providing adequate protein in the diets of vegetarians and vegans, they have many other benefits. Consuming them as part of a meal will reduce glucose levels after that meal, as well as after subsequent meals. (This benefit is lost if the grain is highly refined.) Eating chickpeas or kidney beans – which some people call pulses – at lunch will lower your glycaemic index levels at dinnertime, too. Have them at dinner and your glucose levels will remain low throughout the night.

Beans and grains are a very cheap and handy pantry staple. You can buy different varieties and forms, and they are easily stored dry for several months.

There is a misconception that beans and grains are hard to cook. That's not true. Prepare a batch once or twice a week to be refrigerated and used as you need them. Some, like chickpeas and fava and borlotti beans, need to be soaked for 24 hours before you cook them. Most, however, can be added to a saucepan of boiling water whenever you are doing some cooking and have a hotplate free. You'll need at least three cups of water for every cup of beans or lentils you're cooking because they soak up lots of moisture. Keep an eye on them as they're simmering away to ensure they don't dry out and burn (just add some more water to the saucepan if the level drops) and skim off any foam that collects on top of the water. Drain the legumes, then once they're cool, add a little salt and place them in the fridge, ready for use. This technique works just as well for whole grains like barley, farro and brown rice.

Cooked legumes and grains are easily added to a salad or soup, providing substance and nutrients. If you're using them in salad, a squeeze of lemon juice improves the flavour and the availability of vitamins and minerals, particularly iron and calcium.

The good oil

You may have heard people talk about the Mediterranean diet, which has been shown to reduce the risk of heart disease, diabetes, certain cancers, depression and other Western illnesses. It follows what would be a traditional diet in Spain or southern Italy, and is loaded with vegetables, whole grains, beans, nuts, fruits and seafood. The diet's principles have been adapted for the way of eating recommended in this book.

Another important element of the Mediterranean diet is extra-virgin olive oil, one of the healthiest and most nutritionally dense condiments available. See if you can find cold-pressed extra-virgin olive oil – it is better quality and has a nicer flavour – when you're shopping. Olive oil should always be consumed within 12 to 14 months of pressing, so check the batch and bottling date.

Use good olive oil when roasting, sautéing or in dressings and drizzled over raw or cooked vegetables. You can have too much of a good thing, though. It's important to remember that one tablespoon of olive oil has about 120 calories. Overconsumption without adequate physical activity can lead to weight gain, which may counteract the beneficial effects of olive oil's polyphenols on inflammation and oxidative stress. Excess weight and abdominal fat can negatively impact chronic inflammation, oxidative stress, insulin sensitivity and overall metabolic health, potentially outweighing the health benefits of olive oil and a healthy vegetarian diet.

Nuts and seeds

These tiny nutritional powerhouses are an essential part of our diets and should not be overlooked. They are particularly high in amino acids, fatty acids, dietary fibre and a variety of vitamins and minerals. Apart from eating a serve as a healthy snack, you can add nuts and seeds to salads or blend them into smoothies, sauces and dips.

There's growing scientific evidence that eating a serving of nuts five times a week can cut your chances of developing heart disease by 40 to 60 per cent. A serving is equivalent to a small handful. For reference, that's about 20 almonds, nine walnuts, 30 pistachios, 15 cashews or about two tablespoons of pine nuts.

When shopping, always buy organic raw nuts still in their shells. Some seeds, such as pine nuts, sunflower seeds, watermelon seeds and pumpkin seeds, need to be soaked overnight before you can eat them.

If you haven't already, you should consider adding chia seeds to your diet. They are one of the best plant-origin sources of omega-3 fatty acids (usually found in fish and seafood) and are a rich source of calcium, phosphorous, zinc and copper. Many people like to consume them at breakfast because they also can leave you feeling full for a long time.

What about superfoods?

If you've ever bought supplements online or googled a health question, your social media algorithm is likely to feed you advertisements about miracle powders made from magical ingredients harvested from hundreds of metres below the sea or deep in the Amazon rainforest. If you're eating in the way we propose in this book, whether it includes some or no meat, seafood or animal products, you'll already be getting a full complement of vitamins, minerals, antioxidants and just about every other nutrient your body needs. In fact, many of the foods we recommend – dark green, leafy vegetables; legumes, berries, nuts and seeds – are superfoods in their own right. There's no need to spend hundreds of dollars on supplements.

Set up your kitchen for plant-based success

Before embarking on any new eating plan or making healthy changes, it's wise to start with a clean slate. Begin by going through your pantry and fridge to remove any items that might tempt you to stray from your goals. Clearing out these less healthy options will help you create a space that supports your journey toward a plant-focused lifestyle.

Here's what you should get rid of:

- **Sodas and sweetened drinks:** This includes even those labelled as diet or zero-calorie. These drinks are often loaded with high-fructose corn syrup or artificial sweeteners.

- **Packaged snacks:** Sweet or savory, these snacks are typically high refined carbs and unhealthy fats, sugars and sodium.

- **Mass-produced packaged breads and buns:** These are often made with refined flours, added sugars and preservatives.

- **Instant noodles and soups:** These quick-fix meals are usually high in sodium, unhealthy fats, and lack the nutrients your body needs.

- **Frozen or shelf-stable ready meals:** Often laden with preservatives, artificial flavours and unhealthy fats.

- **Industrialised confectionery and desserts:** These include cookies, cakes and other sweets that are high in sugars, saturated or partially hydrogenated fats, and often contain artificial ingredients.

- **Candy and chocolates:** Loaded with sugar and artificial ingredients.

- **Other ultra-processed foods:** Anything made primarily from sugar, oils, fats and substances not commonly used in homemade cooking, such as hydrogenated oils, modified starches and protein isolates, should be eliminated.

In their place, stock your pantry with legumes, whole grains, dried herbs and spices, extra-virgin olive oil, nuts and seeds.

The same goes for your fridge. Here, you'll store fresh fruit and vegetables, avocados, fresh herbs and chillies, and, if you're still eating them, free-range eggs, low-fat yoghurt, fresh fish and cheese.

Should you include plant-based meat substitutes in your diet?

The rapid growth of plant-based meat substitutes in recent years warrants a degree of caution. While these products offer a promising alternative to traditional meat, many are heavily processed and can contain a range of additives. Often, they include added sugars, saturated fats, salt, as well as stabilisers and preservatives to enhance flavour, texture and shelf life.

These ingredients, while common in processed foods, can contribute to health concerns if consumed in large amounts. Added sugars and saturated fats, for instance, are linked to various health issues, including increased risk of cardiovascular disease. Excessive salt intake is associated with hypertension, stroke and other health problems.

Moreover, stabilisers and preservatives, although they help maintain the product's quality and safety, can sometimes have long-term health implications. It's important for consumers to be mindful of the nutritional profiles of these products and to balance their diets with whole, minimally processed foods.

Plant-centric eating and fasting

There are potential benefits to fasting – you just need to do it properly. The 5:2 diet, where you eat normally for five days and drastically cut calories for two, has become a popular way to lose or maintain weight.

If you're new to plant-based eating, using those two 'fasting' days for creating tasty, nutritious vegan or vegetarian meals can be an excellent stepping stone to adopting it as a larger lifestyle choice.

The biggest mistake people make during the other five days of the week is assuming that 'normal' eating means consuming anything you like, including fast food or junk food with little to no nutritional value. To make the most of those two fasting days, the 'normal' food days should consist of mostly vegetables, legumes and whole grains, plus some seafood, eggs and dairy (if you're still consuming animal products), nuts, seeds, good oils (avocado and extra-virgin olive oil) and fruit.

If you only eat vegetarian or vegan meals during your two fasting days, there is no need to get out the scales or count calories. If you choose a majority of non-starchy vegetables – salad greens, carrots, tomatoes, cauliflower, eggplant, beetroot – and add some beans, you will feel full, be maximising your fibre intake (excellent for your gut health) and consuming few calories. You can even add a little dressing made from extra-virgin olive oil, lemon, vinegar, pepper and spices for flavour without adding many calories.

Another method of fasting you might like to try is 16:8. This involves restricting your daily food intake to the eight hours between 7 am and 2 pm. This involves eating a hearty breakfast, good lunch and a light dinner (usually soup or vegetables). You can do this every day or every second day.

One of our studies showed you can reduce your calorie intake by about 20 per cent every week by replacing lunch and dinner twice a week with a big plate of non-starchy vegetables.

What is most important, regardless of the form of fasting you undertake, is the quality of the food you consume. Eating highly processed foods, refined grains or sugar-sweetened drinks will have detrimental effects on your overall health and can increase the chance of developing chronic illnesses. Choose good quality, real foods.

the fontana healthy longevity code

1. **Reduce waistline & increase skeletal muscle mass**

   - Take action to reduce your waist circumference with regular endurance exercise training and moderate calorie restriction, ensuring you consume the right amount of nutrient-rich calories for optimal functioning.

   - Enhance or maintain muscle mass with strength-training exercises two to three times per week.

2. **Adopt a predominantly plant-centric diet**

   - Staple foods should include a diverse selection of vegetables, minimally processed whole grains, legumes, seeds, nuts and low-glycaemic fruits. Refined carbohydrates should be avoided.

   - Eat mostly proteins from plants (legumes, whole grains and nuts). Consider fish, seafood and low-fat dairy as secondary sources of protein to provide essential nutrients like vitamin B12, zinc and omega-3 fatty acids. If consuming meat or poultry, choose lean cuts sparingly and avoid processed meats.

   - Select cold-pressed extra-virgin olive oil in moderation for cooking and dressing.

   Avoid animal fats (butter, cream), tropical oils (coconut, palm) and partially hydrogenated fats.

   - Steer clear of ultra-processed foods and sweetened beverages, which are rich in 'empty' calories, sugars and unhealthy fats. Use minimal salt in cooking; opt for iodised salt to support thyroid health.

3. **Intermittent fasting and time-restricted eating**

   - If overweight, aim to stop eating when you are 80 per cent full. Once or twice a week, consume only non-starchy vegetable and legume salads.

   - Focus on consuming all meals within an 8 – 10-hour window each day, avoiding snacks between meals. Practice mindful eating, ideally shared with your family or friends.

4. **Engage in daily physical activity**

   - Dedicate at least 30 – 60 minutes each day to physical exercise, alternating between aerobic, strength, flexibility and balance workouts.

   - Minimise sitting time by moving frequently throughout the day, and incorporate enjoyable, social activities with friends into your daily routine.

5. Avoid or limit alcohol consumption

- If you do not currently drink alcohol, it is best not to start.

- If you choose to consume alcohol, keep your intake minimal to reduce the risk of cancer, atrial fibrillation, heart disease and brain aging.

6. Avoid smoking and vaping

- Refrain from using any form of tobacco, including e-cigarettes and vaping.

7. Prioritise quality sleep

- Set a bedtime early enough to ensure you get 7 – 9 hours of sleep each night.

- Maintain a consistent sleep schedule, create a sleep-conducive environment, and turn off electronic devices at least 30 minutes before bedtime.

8. Nourish and protect your mind

- Reduce mental stress through mindful meditation and slow deep-breathing exercises.

- Engage your mind daily by learning new skills or participating in artistic activities to enhance cognitive function and brain health.

- Embrace a lifelong commitment to self-awareness and personal growth, continually seeking new knowledge, experiences and perspectives for intellectual and spiritual vitality, and human flourishing.

9. Cultivate friendship, altruism and compassion

- Foster strong relationships with family and friends through empathetic communication and forgiveness.

- Engage in daily acts of altruism and compassion to strengthen neural pathways associated with peace and wellbeing.

10. Minimise pollution exposure and connect with nature

- Limit your exposure to pollutants, including air, water and noise pollution.

- Immerse yourself in nature whenever possible. **Exercising in unpolluted environments, especially in parks and wooded areas, offers significant cardioprotective and psychological benefits.**

Adapted from Cagigas ML, Twigg SM, Fontana L. Ten tips for promoting cardiometabolic health and slowing cardiovascular aging. Eur Heart J. 2024;45(13):1094-1097.

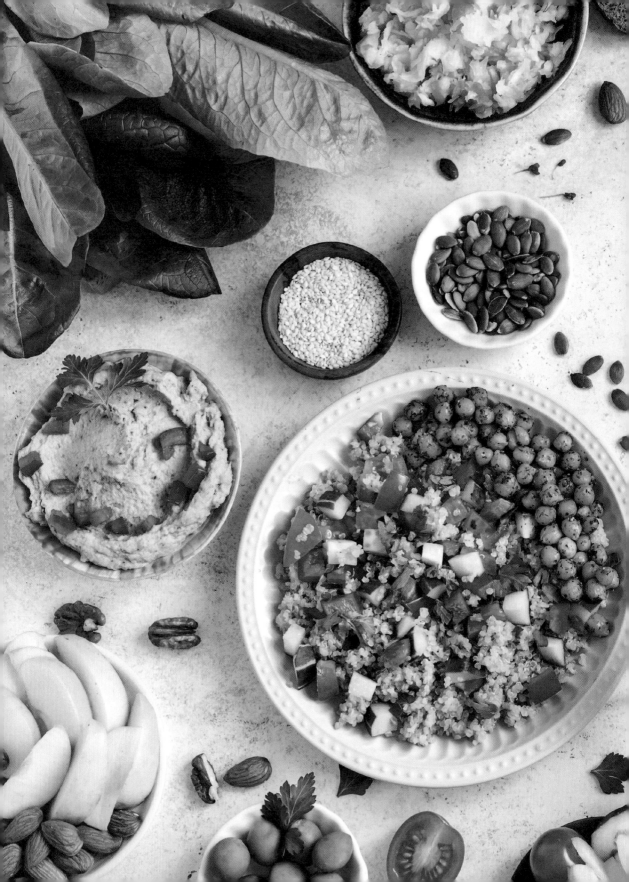

RECIPES

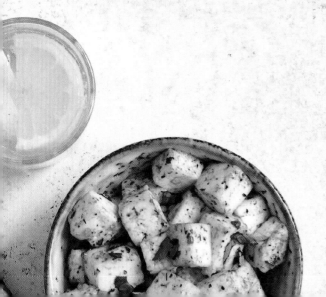

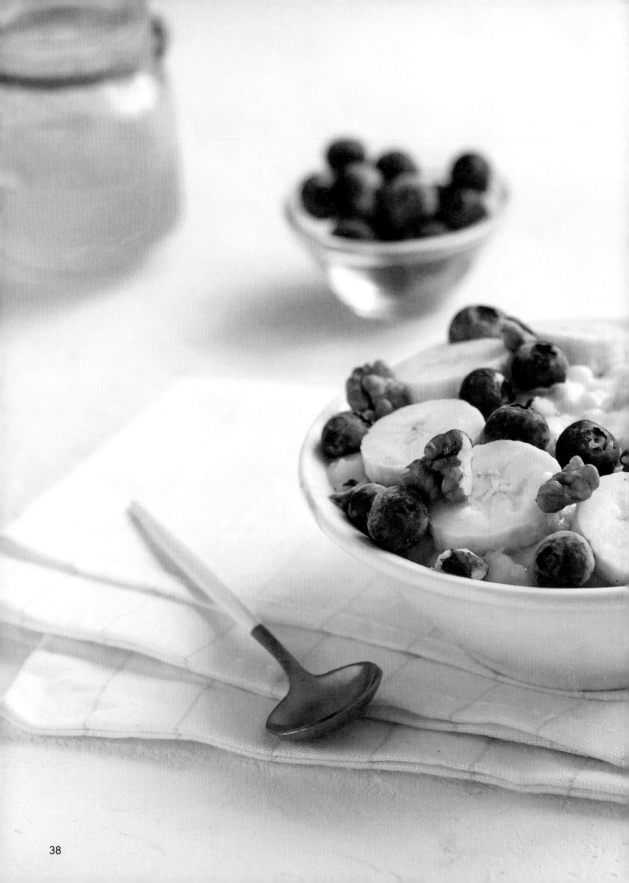

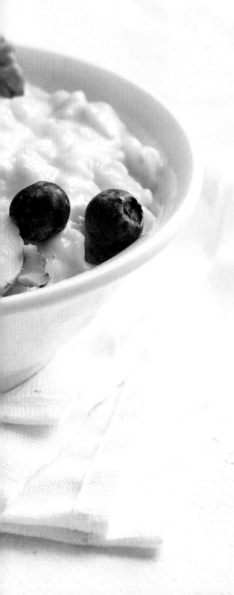

Breakfast

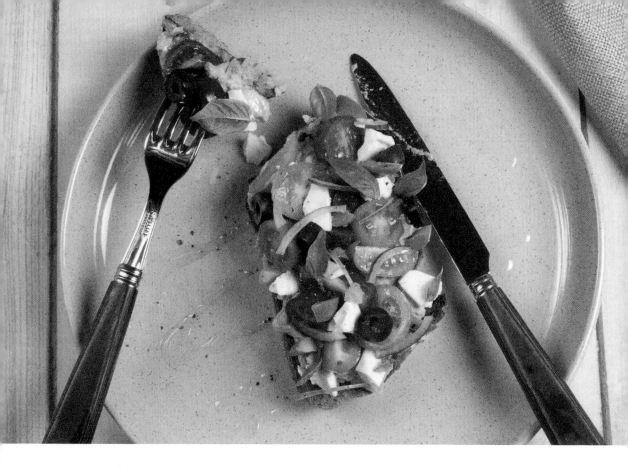

Bruschetta with avocado, olives, tomatoes, feta and basil

SERVES 4

4 slices wholemeal sourdough bread

2 avocados

½ small red onion, thinly sliced

16 kalamata olives, pitted and sliced

200 g (7 oz) heirloom cherry tomatoes, quartered

50 g (1¾ oz) Danish feta, crumbled

1 cup basil leaves, loosely packed

juice of 1 lemon to taste

salt and pepper to taste

2 tablespoons extra virgin olive oil

Toast the bread in a toaster or under the grill.

In the meantime, scoop out the flesh of the avocados into a bowl, and season with salt, pepper, lemon juice and extra virgin olive oil. Crush the avocado into a chunky paste using a fork and spread onto the toast. Top with the remaining ingredients, and season further with salt, pepper, lemon juice and olive oil.

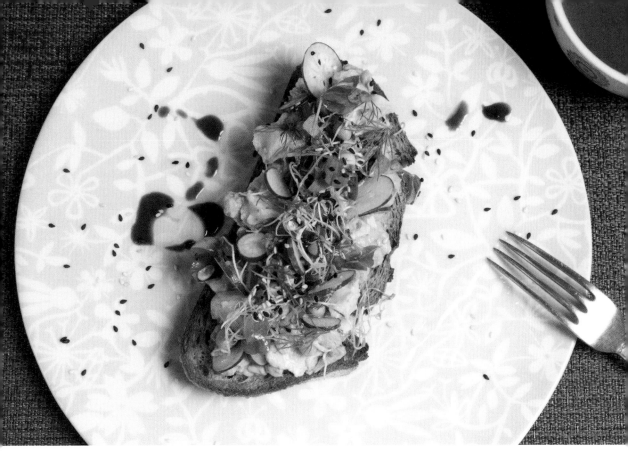

Bruschetta with avocado, cashew cheese and sprout salad

SERVES 4

2 small avocados

1 lime, juiced

4 radishes, thinly sliced

2 cups mixed sprouts (e.g., mung bean,
  alfalfa, snow pea)

2 spring onions, thinly sliced

½ cup dill leaves, finely chopped

1½ tablespoons tamari

2 tablespoons extra virgin olive oil

4 slices wholemeal sourdough bread

80 g (2¾ oz) cashew cheese (or feta), crumbled

2 tablespoons sesame seeds, toasted

salt and pepper to taste

Deseed the avocados and scoop out the flesh.
Place the flesh in a bowl and mash with a fork.
Add half the lime juice and season with salt
and pepper. Set aside.

Place the radish, sprouts, spring onions and dill
in a separate bowl and gently mix. Dress with
the tamari, olive oil and remaining lime juice.

In the meantime, toast the bread in a toaster or
under the grill. Spread the mashed avocado on
the toast, top with cashew cheese, a handful
of the sprout salad and sesame seeds. Drizzle
with more tamari and olive oil if desired.

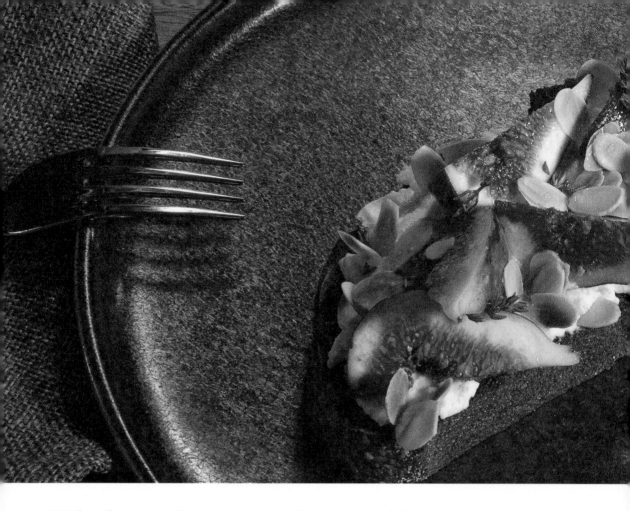

Wholemeal toast with ricotta, figs, almonds and thyme honey

SERVES 4

4 slices wholemeal sourdough bread

6 ripe figs

250 g (9 oz) ricotta

35 g (1¼ oz) almond flakes, toasted

20 g (¾ oz) thyme honey (see below)

FOR THE THYME HONEY
300 g (10½ oz) honey

15 g (½ oz) thyme sprigs

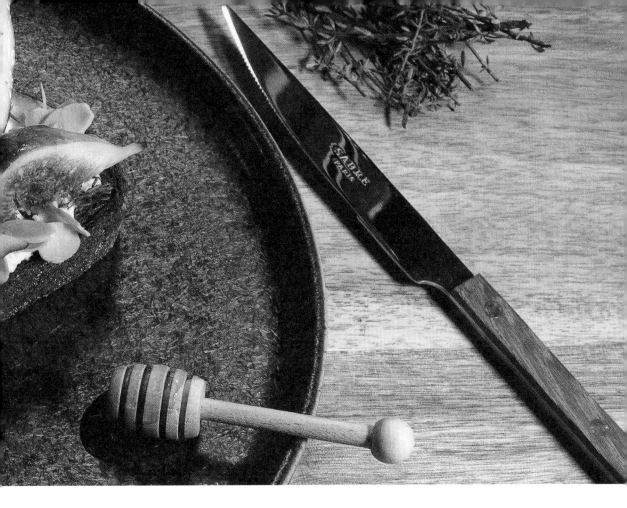

To make the thyme honey, put a third of the honey with the thyme in a microwave jug. Warm until hot and fully liquid. If using a small saucepan, warm the honey and thyme over a medium heat just until simmering. Cool to room temperature, then combine with the rest of the honey and set aside to infuse for 24 hours or more. Remove the thyme when the honey is well flavoured. Store and use like ordinary honey.

Toast the bread in a toaster or under the grill. While the bread is toasting, quarter the figs.

Spread the ricotta on the toasted sourdough. Arrange six pieces of fig on each slice and scatter with the almonds. Drizzle with the thyme honey.

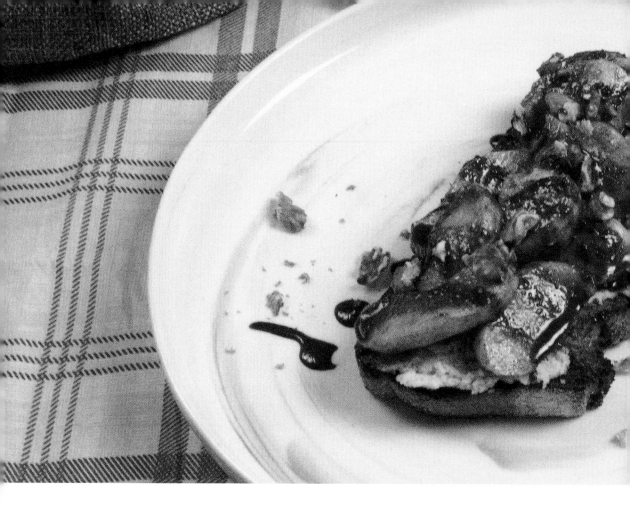

Wholemeal toast with hazelnut cocoa butter and baked apples

SERVES 4

3 red eating apples

1 teaspoon honey

1 tablespoon lemon juice

10 g (¼ oz) vanilla paste

½ teaspoon ground cinnamon

4 slices wholemeal sourdough bread

160 g (5½ oz) hazelnut cocoa butter

20 g (¾ oz) toasted walnuts

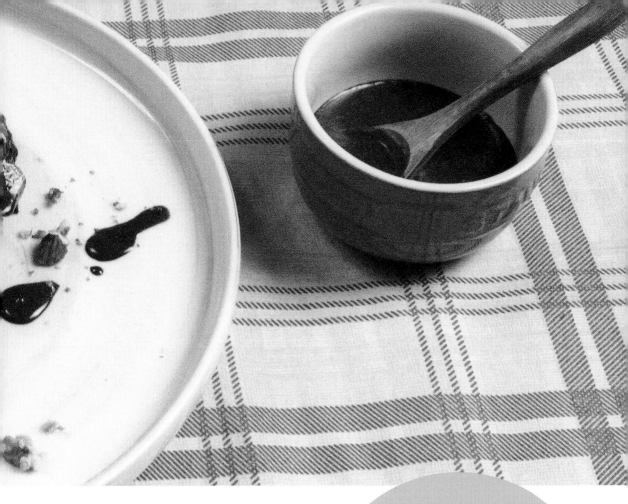

Preheat the oven to 170°C (340°F).

Peel and core the apples and cut them into eighths. Place in a bowl with the honey, lemon, vanilla and cinnamon. Mix well until all the apple pieces are evenly coated. Place onto a lined baking sheet. Bake for 10 minutes, then turn the apple pieces over and bake for a further 10 minutes, raising the heat to 230°C (450°F). Remove once well coloured and still intact. While the apples are cooling, toast the bread.

Spread each slice of toast with hazelnut butter, arrange the apples over the top and sprinkle with chopped walnuts.

Nuts

Nuts (with the exception of macadamias) are low in saturated fats, and rich in the cardio-protective monounsaturated and polyunsaturated fats.

They are rich in soluble fibre that may help reduce blood pressure and the absorption of cholesterol in our intestine.

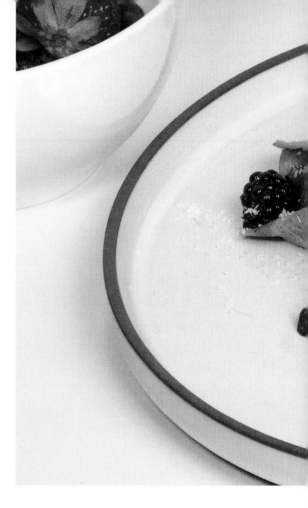

Crepes with bbq pineapple, berries and spiced yoghurt

SERVES 4

FOR THE FILLING
100 g (3½ oz) raisins (golden)

200 ml (7 fl oz) hot tea of choice (green, black, herbal)

1 large pineapple

300 g (10½ oz) low-fat Greek yoghurt

40 g (1½ oz) date paste (page 184)

10 g (¼ oz) vanilla paste

½ teaspoon ground cinnamon

FOR THE BATTER
130 g (4½ oz) wholemeal flour

200 g (7 oz) unsweetened non-dairy milk of choice (soy, nut, oat)

100 ml (3½ fl oz) water

2 eggs

10 g (¼ oz) vanilla paste

2 teaspoons honey

1 pinch salt

25 ml (¾ fl oz) extra virgin olive oil

2 teaspoons wattleseed (optional)

olive oil, additional for cooking

TO SERVE
mixed fresh berries

handful mint leaves, torn

4 macadamia nuts, very finely chopped

Soak the raisins in the hot tea and leave for at least an hour. Drain when plump and set the raisins aside in a medium-sized bowl.

Meanwhile, peel, core and cut the pineapple into 1½ cm (½ in) slices. Heat a grill or BBQ to high (or use a grill pan). Place the pineapple on the grill, turning as it browns. What you are looking for is caramelisation but no black burn marks. Once all the pineapple is grilled, set aside to cool. When the pineapple is cool enough to work with, dice and mix with the raisins. Set aside until needed.

For the spiced yoghurt, combine the yoghurt with the date paste, vanilla and cinnamon.

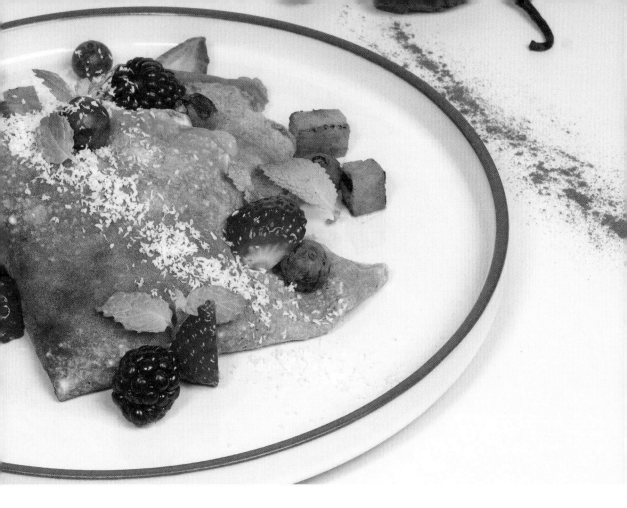

To make the crepes, place the flour, milk, water, eggs, vanilla, honey, salt, olive oil and wattleseed (if using) in a food processor or blender and process until a batter forms. Don't overmix. Rest batter in the fridge for 30 minutes.

Heat a 23 cm (9 in) crepe pan over medium–high heat. Pour ½ teaspoon of olive oil in the pan and use some kitchen paper to spread the oil across the base of the pan, leaving just a thin film. When the pan is hot pour 50 ml (1¾ fl oz or about ¼ cup) of batter and tilt the pan to swirl the batter around to form a thin, even layer. Using a spatula gently lift the crepe once the edges are coloured to check if it has set and browned slightly on the

bottom. Flip the crepe and cook for a further 20–30 seconds. Place the crepe on a warm plate and set aside. Repeat the process, stacking the crepes on top of one another, until all the batter has been used.

To assemble, place a spoonful of yoghurt and a spoonful of the pineapple and raisin mix in each crepe and roll into a cylinder shape. Serve with fresh berries, mint and nuts.

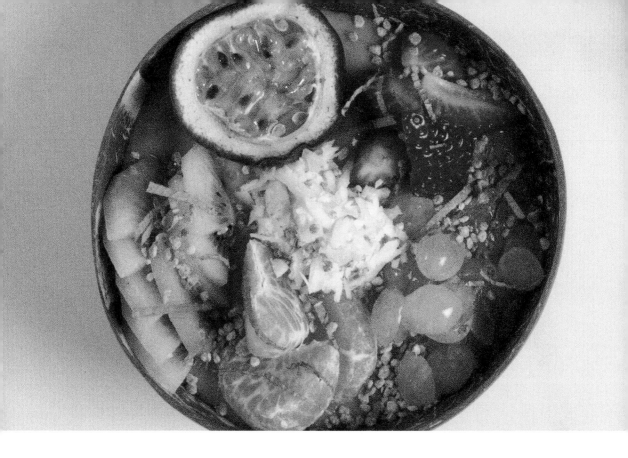

Tropical smoothie bowl with bee pollen and brazil nuts

SERVES 4

FOR THE SMOOTHIE
1 large mango

¼ large papaya

1 carrot, peeled

½ teaspoon fresh ginger

2 frozen ripe bananas, chopped

FOR THE TOPPING
1 mandarin, segmented

2 kiwifruit, peeled and sliced

2 passionfruit, halved

2 cups grapes

6 large strawberries, quartered

8 Brazil nuts, chopped

½ cup mint leaves, thinly sliced

4 tablespoons bee pollen

For the smoothie, peel, deseed and dice the mango and papaya. Grate the carrot and ginger. Transfer to a medium bowl and refrigerate while you prepare the topping ingredients.

When ready, combine the chilled smoothie ingredients and the frozen bananas in a blender. Process to a smooth, thick consistency. Pour into four serving bowls. Top with the fruit and nuts, and garnish with the mint and bee pollen.

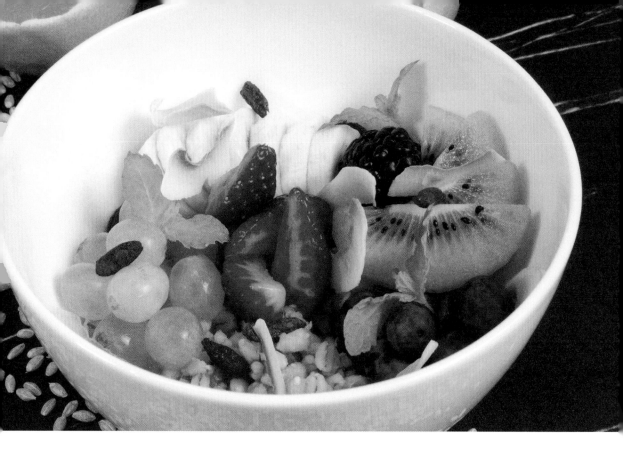

Morning barley fruit salad

SERVES 4

160 g (5½ oz) pearl barley

40 g (1½ oz) almonds, crushed

4 oranges, juiced

4 strawberries, hulled and sliced

8 blackberries

75 g (2¾ oz) blueberries

2 handfuls grapes

1 banana, sliced

1 kiwifruit, peeled and sliced

4 tablespoons coconut flakes, toasted

2 tablespoons goji berries

½ cup mint leaves

Ahead of time, bring a medium-sized saucepan of water to a boil. Add the barley and a pinch of salt and simmer for around 30 minutes or until cooked. Drain and place in a covered bowl in the fridge to chill.

Prepare the fruit toppings. When ready to serve, divide the barley and almonds between four wide bowls, pour over the orange juice and mix well. Arrange the fruit on top with the coconut, goji berries and mint as desired.

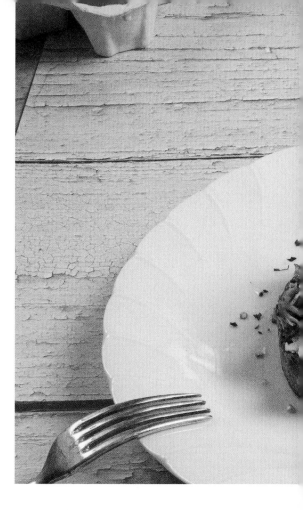

Rye bruschetta with ricotta, broccoli, chilli, poached egg and parmesan

SERVES 4

400 g (14 oz) broccoli

1 garlic clove, finely chopped

1½ tablespoons extra virgin olive oil

¾ tablespoon smoked paprika

60 g (2 oz) almond flakes

2 tablespoons white vinegar

4 eggs

4 slices rye sourdough

120 g (4½ oz) ricotta

30 g (1 oz) grated parmesan

juice of 1 lemon to taste

salt and pepper

chilli flakes to taste

Preheat the oven to 230°C (450°F).

Meanwhile, break down the broccoli into small florets. Combine in a bowl with the garlic, olive oil, paprika and season with salt and pepper. Mix well to coat each piece of broccoli. Transfer to a lined baking sheet and bake for 15 minutes, giving it a toss every 5 minutes. We are after slightly charred and crispy florets. Remove from the oven and lower the oven to 160°C (320°F). When cool enough to handle, roughly chop the broccoli into popcorn-sized chunks. Transfer to a bowl and keep warm.

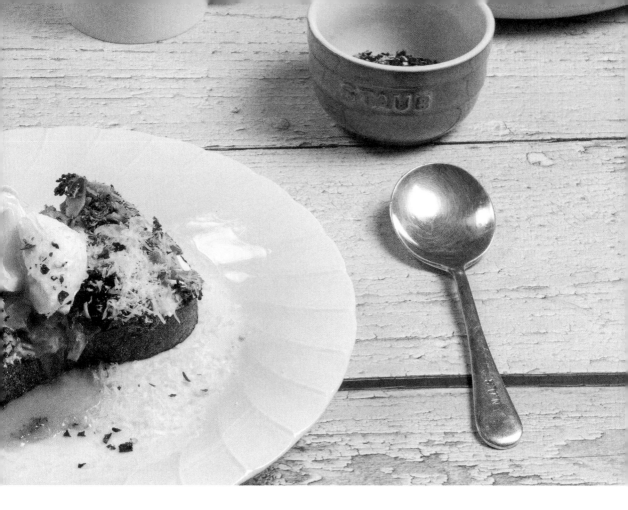

Place the almond flakes in a single layer on a clean baking tray, and toast until lightly golden (approximately 8 minutes). Be careful not to burn them.

Half-fill a medium-sized saucepan with water and place over a high heat, add the vinegar and bring to a rolling boil. Once boiling, reduce to a simmer. Carefully break the eggs into a small bowl. Swirl the simmering water with a slotted spoon, before gently sliding all four eggs in. You may need to swirl the water again to stop the eggs sticking to the bottom. Cook for 2–3 minutes or until the whites are set and the yolks are still runny.

Meanwhile, toast the bread. Divide the ricotta between the slices of toast and spread to cover the whole slice. Dress the broccoli with lemon juice to taste and extra salt and pepper if needed. Arrange across the toast. Top each slice with a poached egg, parmesan, almonds and chilli flakes.

Dosa with kale, roast tomatoes, raita and fried egg

SERVES 4

FOR THE DOSA
900 ml (30½ fl oz) water

330 g (11½ oz) brown rice

190 g (6½ oz) red lentils

1 teaspoon fenugreek, ground

1 teaspoon cumin seeds

½ teaspoon turmeric

1 teaspoon salt

extra virgin olive oil

FOR THE FILLING
12 cherry tomatoes

220 g (8 oz) kale

3 French eschalots

2 garlic cloves

1 tablespoon extra virgin olive oil

½ teaspoon Madras curry powder

½ tablespoons lime juice

salt to taste

4 eggs (optional)

coriander (cilantro) leaves

FOR THE RAITA
7 mint leaves

1 small green chilli, deseeded

½ Lebanese cucumber

¼ teaspoon ground cumin

200 g (7 oz) low-fat Greek yoghurt

salt and pepper to taste

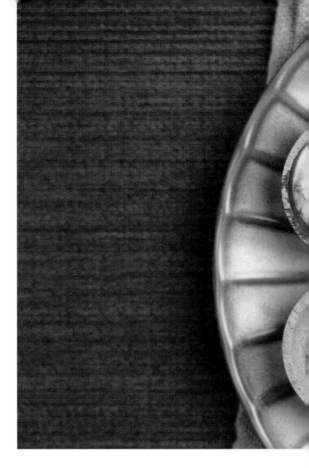

Wash the rice and lentils, then soak in plenty of water for about 5–6 hours. Drain well and combine with the remaining dosa ingredients in a food processor. Blend until you reach a creamy consistency. Place the batter in a bowl, cover and leave at room temperature for fermentation overnight (10–12 hours).

The next day, preheat the oven to 150°C (300°F). In a small bowl, toss the cherry tomatoes with a little olive oil, salt and pepper. Place on a lined baking tray and roast for 20 minutes, until soft but still holding their shape. Set aside.

In the meantime, prepare the raita. Finely chop the mint and chilli. Finely grate the cucumber and squeeze all the water from it using a cloth or in a sieve. Combine the mint, chilli, cucumber and cumin with the yoghurt in a bowl. Season

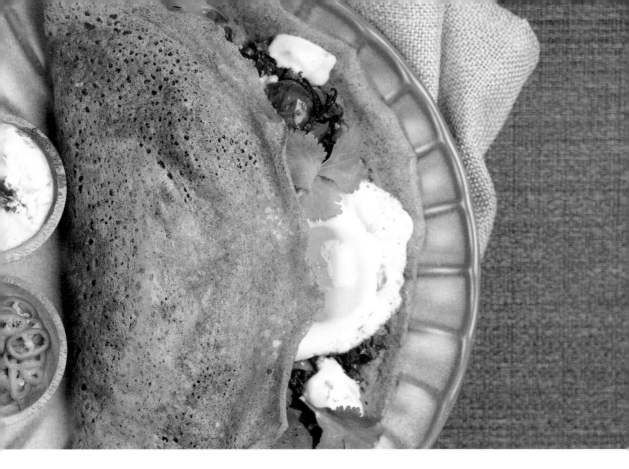

to taste and mix well. Cover and refrigerate until ready to use.

Prepare the kale by removing the central stems from the leaves. Wash and dry the leaves well and cut into 5 mm (¼ inch) slices. Finely slice the eschalots and mince the garlic.

Place a large frying pan on high heat with 1 tablespoon of olive oil. Once hot add the kale and eschalot. Toss for about 1–2 minutes or until almost wilted. Add the garlic, curry powder, lime juice and salt and continue cooking for a further minute. Remove from the heat and keep warm.

To cook the dosa, heat a 30 cm (11¾ in) non-stick frying pan over a high heat. Very lightly oil the pan with a few drops of oil spread with a paper towel. Once hot, pour

½ cup of batter into the pan. Tilt the pan and swirl the batter to evenly coat the base. Cook until it starts to come away at the edges and the top is set. Flip the dosa, cook for another 5–10 seconds and place on a serving plate. Repeat, making a stack, using up all the batter. Cook the eggs, if using, in the same frying pan.

To serve, divide the kale mix and cherry tomatoes amongst the dosa, top with raita and coriander leaves. Add a fried egg (if using), fold the dosa closed and enjoy.

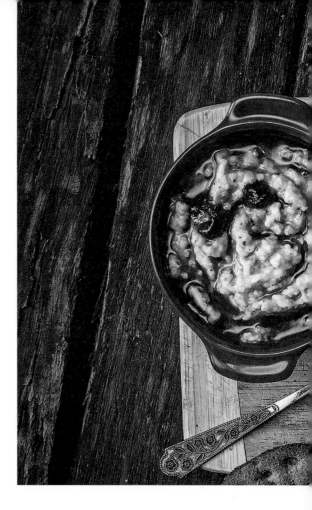

Cocoa, oat and hemp seed porridge with poached berries and walnuts

SERVES 4

FOR THE PORRIDGE

250 g (9 oz) steel cut oats

250 ml (8½ fl oz) milk of choice (soy, nut, oat)

2 very ripe bananas

½ cup hemp seeds

1½ tablespoons cocoa powder

50 g (1¾ oz) toasted walnuts, crushed

FOR THE BERRIES

225 g (8 oz) frozen mixed berries

20 g (¾ oz) honey

4 g (⅛ oz) vanilla extract

1 tablespoon lemon juice

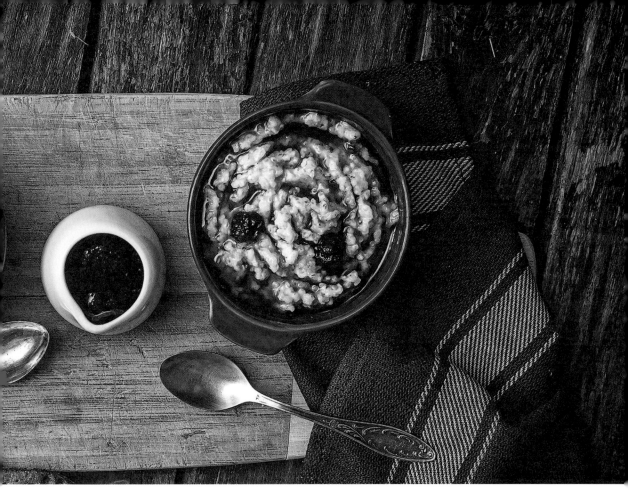

The night before, soak the oats in 450 ml (15¼ fl oz) of water and place in the fridge overnight. The next day, transfer the soaked oats to a saucepan, add the milk and bring to a simmer over a medium heat. Turn down the heat and continue to simmer for 25–30 minutes or until thick and cooked, stirring every 5 minutes to avoid sticking.

For the berries, place all the ingredients in a small saucepan and bring to the boil. Then remove the berries using a slotted spoon and set aside in a small bowl. Simmer the remaining liquid in the saucepan until it has reduced to a syrup. Cool the syrup slightly and return the berries to the pan. Set aside until ready to use.

Place the bananas in a small bowl with the hemp seeds and cocoa powder and mash well with a fork. Once the porridge is cooked, remove from the heat and fold the banana mixture through. Serve the porridge topped with the berries and walnuts.

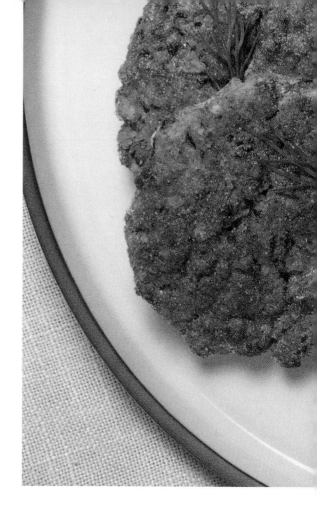

Chickpea and zucchini fritters with broad bean and herb salad

SERVES 4

FOR THE FRITTERS

100 g (3½ oz) cooked chickpeas

2 medium zucchini (courgette)

½ onion, finely diced

100 g (3½ oz) cooked quinoa

1 garlic clove, minced

½ teaspoon ground cumin

½ teaspoon ground coriander

½ teaspoon smoked paprika

¼ teaspoon salt

black pepper to taste

2 teaspoons nutritional yeast

1 tablespoon chopped parsley

chickpea flour, to dust

1 tablespoon extra virgin olive oil

FOR THE SALAD

2 spring onions

1 long red chilli, deseeded

2 cups cooked broad beans (fresh or frozen)

1 handful mint leaves, finely chopped

1 handful coriander (cilantro) leaves, finely chopped

½ lemon, juiced

½ tablespoon extra virgin olive oil

salt and pepper to taste

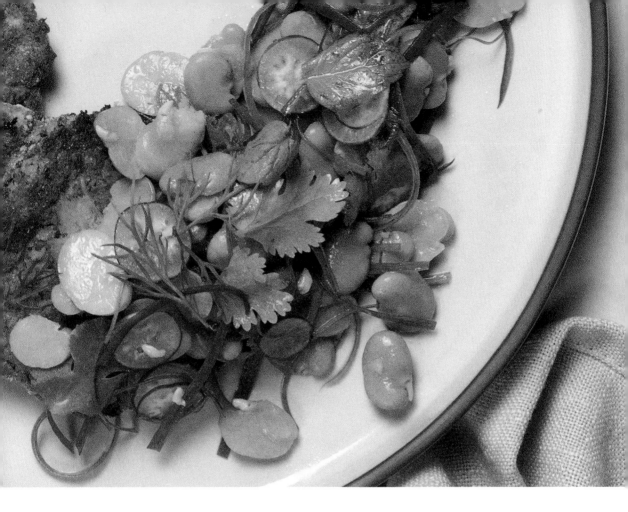

Preheat the oven to 200°C (400°F). In a food processor, blend the cooked chickpeas to a paste and transfer to a large bowl. Grate the zucchini and squeeze in a cloth to remove the liquid, then add to the chickpeas. Fold in all the remaining fritter ingredients except the chickpea flour. Mix well until everything comes together enough to form into balls. If the mix is too dry and crumbly, add a little water or plant-based milk.

Divide the mix into eight balls and press down gently to form fritters. Dust each fritter lightly in chickpea flour. Lightly oil a baking tray large enough to fit all the fritters and place it in the hot oven to heat up (about 1 minute). Place the fritters on the tray and bake until golden underneath, about 12 minutes. Gently turn them over and repeat on the other side.

Meanwhile, to make the salad, thinly slice the spring onions and chilli. Transfer to a serving bowl with the rest of the ingredients, dress with lemon juice and olive oil. Toss well and season to taste. Divide the fritters between four serving plates and serve with the broad bean salad.

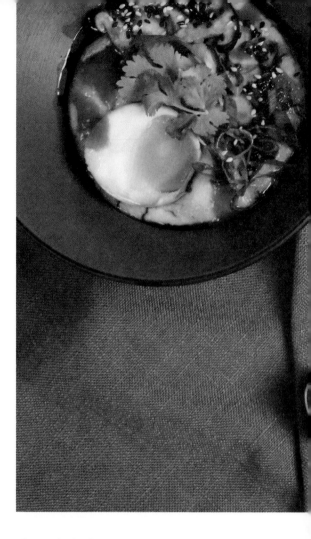

Brown rice porridge with jammy egg, shiitake and fermented chilli

SERVES 4

FOR THE PORRIDGE
1 cup brown rice

2 litres (68 fl oz) water

¼ teaspoon salt

FOR THE TOPPING
3 organic eggs

100 g (3½ oz) tamari

100 ml (3½ fl oz) malt vinegar

1 teaspoon fresh ginger, finely grated

2½ tablespoons extra virgin olive oil

1 tablespoon white sesame seeds

1 tablespoon black sesame seeds

8 shiitake mushrooms, cut into 5 mm (¼ in) slices

2 spring onions, thinly sliced

1 handful coriander (cilantro) leaves, picked

fermented chilli sauce to taste

The night before you plan to serve the porridge, place the brown rice, water and salt in a medium saucepan and bring to the boil. If a foam forms, remove with a spoon and lower the heat. Reduce the heat to very low, cover, and simmer for about 1 hour until cooked. Drain off any excess water, cover, and let stand at room temperature overnight.

Meanwhile, in another saucepan of boiling water, soft boil the eggs for 5–6½ minutes. Remove and cool in ice water. Once the eggs are cold, carefully peel them, leaving them whole, and place in a container just big enough for the eggs or in a ziplock bag. Combine the tamari and vinegar and pour over the eggs so

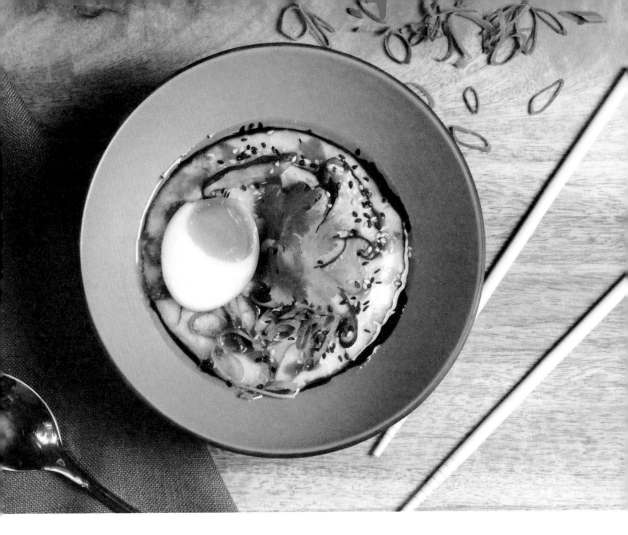

they are submerged in the liquid. Set aside in the fridge overnight.

In the morning, place the rice mixture in a food processor and blend until you reach a creamy porridge consistency. If the mixture is too dry, add a small amount of hot water a little at a time – just enough to give it a slightly soupy consistency. Heat the porridge in a microwave or gently in a saucepan (but don't allow it to stick).

To prepare the toppings, in a small bowl mix together the grated ginger and 2 tablespoons of olive oil. Set aside. Lightly toast the sesame seeds in a hot dry frying pan, then transfer to

a plate to cool. Add the remaining olive oil to the pan and sauté the shiitake mushrooms with 3 tablespoons of water and a pinch of salt. Cook until the liquid has evaporated and the mushrooms have gained good colour.

Divide the hot porridge between four bowls and top with the eggs, mushrooms, spring onions, ginger and sesame seeds. Drizzle over some of the tamari liquid, top with coriander leaves and chilli.

Spiced vegetable quesadilla with black beans

SERVES 4

200 g (7 oz) cooked black beans
1 tablespoon extra virgin olive oil
salt and pepper to taste

FOR THE FILLING
2 cobs fresh sweet corn

2 tomatoes cored, diced

1 red onion, diced

1 zucchini (courgette), diced

1 small red capsicum, diced

1 small yellow capsicum, diced

1 small green capsicum, diced

½ head broccoli, broken into florets

2 garlic cloves, minced

2 teaspoons thyme leaves, chopped

2 teaspoons dried oregano

1 teaspoon smoked paprika

½ teaspoon ground cumin

½ teaspoon ground coriander

½ teaspoon smoked chipotle powder

1 tablespoon extra virgin olive oil

salt and pepper to taste

15 kalamata olives, pitted and sliced

2 tablespoons coriander (cilantro) leaves, chopped

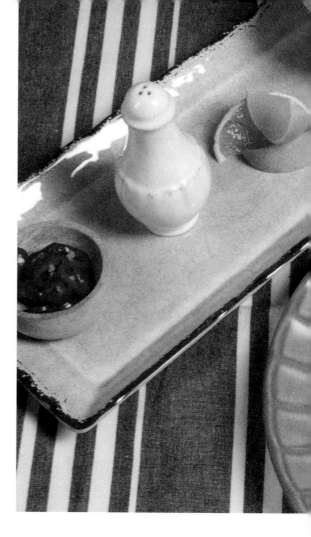

FOR THE YOGHURT SAUCE
200 g (7 oz) low-fat Greek yoghurt

1½ tablespoons coriander (cilantro) leaves, chopped

1 jalapeno, deseeded and chopped

⅓ garlic clove, minced

½ lime, zest and juice

4 large wholemeal tortillas

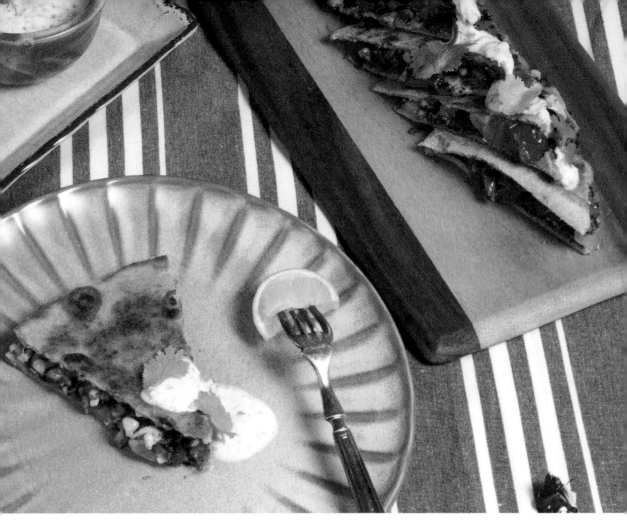

Preheat the oven to 220°C (430°F). Process the black beans in a blender with the olive oil. The consistency should be thick, smooth and creamy. Season to taste and set aside.

Cut the kernels off the corn cobs and place in a deep baking tray. Add all the other filling ingredients except the olives and coriander. Mix well to ensure everything is evenly coated in the oil, herbs and spices. Bake for 20 minutes, mixing a couple of times during the cooking period. In the meantime, mix all the sauce ingredients together in a small bowl.

To assemble, spread 1½ tablespoons of the black bean mix on half of each tortilla. Spoon the vegetable filling on top of that. Scatter with the olives and coriander, then fold the other half of the tortilla over the filling to close.

Very lightly brush one side of the quesadilla with extra virgin olive oil and place on a hot pan or grill and cook until crispy and golden. Lightly oil the other side, then turn the quesadilla over and cook as before. Repeat with all four quesadillas. Cut each quesadilla into four and serve with the yoghurt sauce.

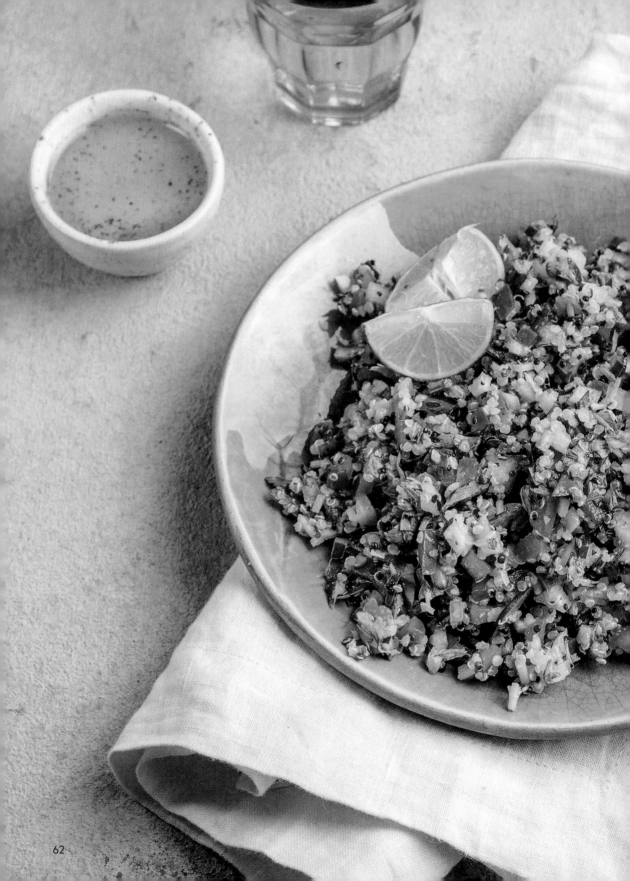

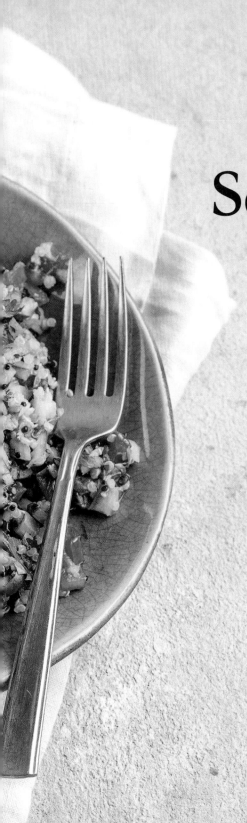

Salads

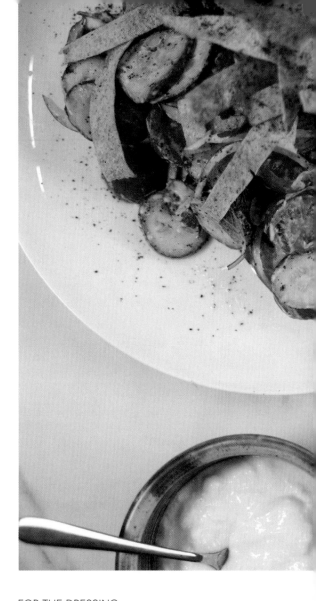

Yoghurt fattoush salad with crispy lebanese bread

SERVES 4

2 wholemeal Lebanese flat-breads

1½ tablespoons extra virgin olive oil

½ tablespoon sumac

½ tablespoon zaatar

½ tablespoon ground fennel seed

400 g (14 oz) cherry tomatoes

5 Lebanese cucumbers

5 radishes

½ red onion

1½ cups parsley leaves, loosely packed

1½ cups mint leaves, loosely packed

salt and pepper to taste

FOR THE DRESSING

60 ml (2 fl oz) lemon juice

120 ml (4 fl oz) extra virgin olive oil

80 g (2¾ oz) low-fat Greek yoghurt

1 teaspoon honey

¼ teaspoon salt

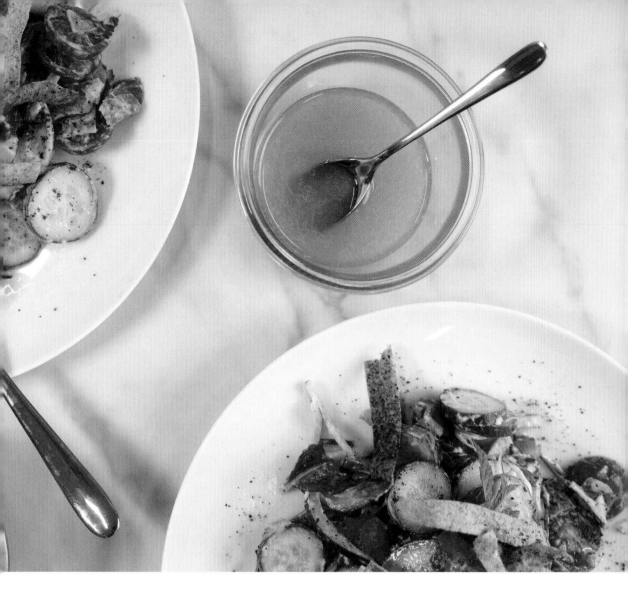

Preheat the oven to 150°C (300°F). Use a knife to separate the two layers of each Lebanese bread to create four rounds. Brush the smooth side of each piece with olive oil. Stack the pieces on top of each other and slice into 1 cm (½ in) strips. Place in a bowl, add the spices and season with a pinch of salt. Mix well and transfer to a baking tray. Bake for 15–30 minutes until dry and crisp.

In the meantime, halve the cherry tomatoes and slice the cucumber into ½ cm (¼ in) thick pieces. Finely slice the radish and onion.

To make the dressing, whisk together all the ingredients in a small bowl until combined.

Combine the vegetables, herbs and half the crisp bread in a salad bowl, dressing to taste and tossing well. Serve topped with the remaining bread.

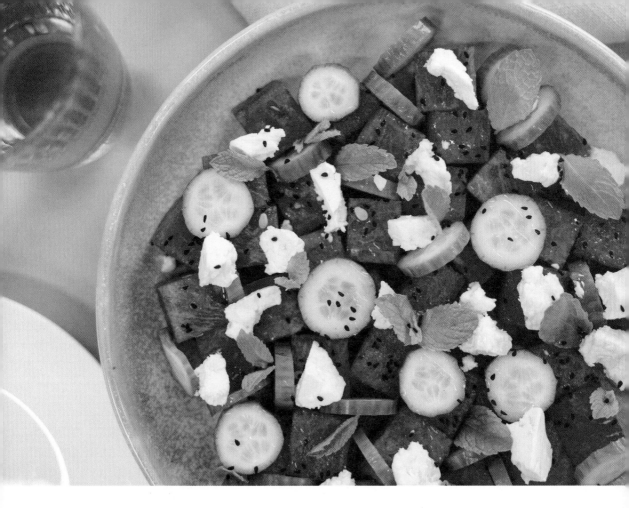

Watermelon salad with feta, mint and cucumber

SERVES 4

½ large watermelon

4 Lebanese cucumbers

120 g (4½ oz) low-fat feta, diced

1 cup mint leaves, loosely packed

1 tablespoon nigella seeds

FOR THE DRESSING

60 ml (2 fl oz) lemon juice

120 ml (4 fl oz) extra virgin olive oil

2 teaspoons honey

¼ teaspoon salt

Peel and dice the watermelon into bite-sized pieces. Slice the Lebanese cucumber into ½ cm (¼ in) rounds. Arrange the watermelon, cucumber, feta and mint on a serving plate. Sprinkle with the nigella seeds.

For the dressing, combine the ingredients in a small bowl to emulsify. Dress the salad to taste and serve.

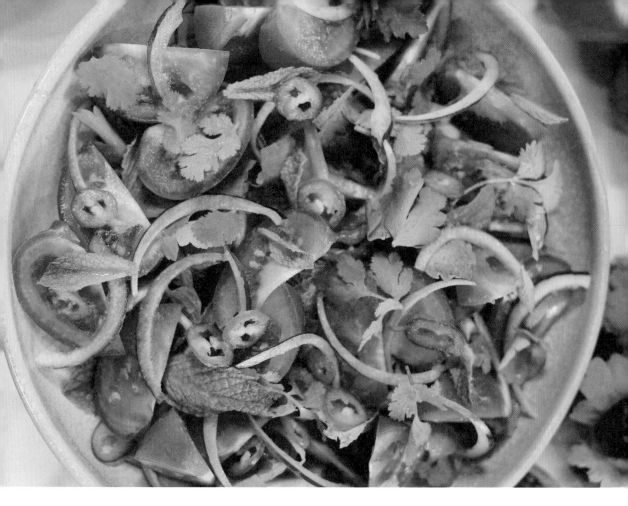

Spicy tomato, herb and cumin salad

SERVES 4

5 large vine-ripened tomatoes

¾ cup mint leaves, loosely packed

¾ cup parsley leaves, loosely packed

¾ cup coriander (cilantro) leaves, loosely packed

½ medium red onion, finely sliced

1 long green chilli, deseeded and finely sliced

FOR THE DRESSING

60 ml (2 fl oz) lemon juice

120 ml (4 fl oz) extra virgin olive oil

2 teaspoons honey

¾ teaspoon ground cumin

¼ teaspoon salt

Wash the tomatoes well and cut into bite-sized wedges. Pick the herbs, leaving them whole. Combine all the salad ingredients in a serving bowl and toss well.

In a separate bowl, whisk the dressing ingredients together to emulsify. Dress the salad to taste and serve.

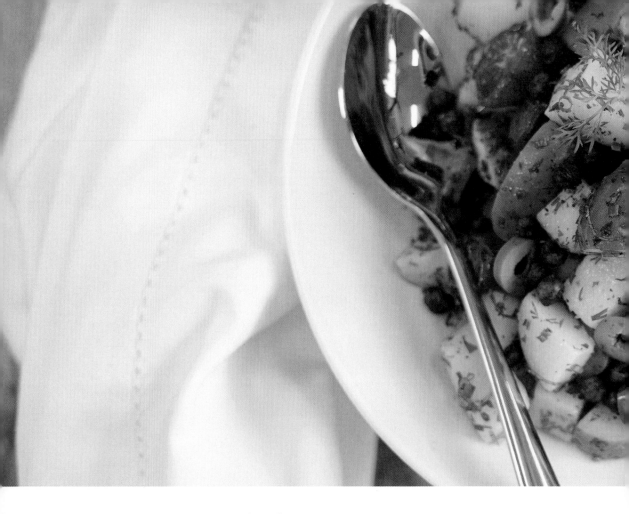

Warm potato salad with semi-dried tomatoes, olives and crispy chickpeas

SERVES 4

250 g (9 oz) cherry tomatoes

½ tablespoon extra virgin olive oil

7 medium sebago potatoes

15 green olives, pitted

1 tablespoon chopped flat-leaf parsley

1 tablespoon chopped mint

1 tablespoon chopped dill

1 tablespoon chopped chives

1 cup Crispy spiced chickpeas (page 185)

salt and pepper

FOR THE DRESSING

60 ml (2 fl oz) white wine vinegar

120 ml (4 fl oz) extra virgin olive oil

30 g (1 oz) Dijon mustard

2 teaspoons honey

¼ teaspoon salt

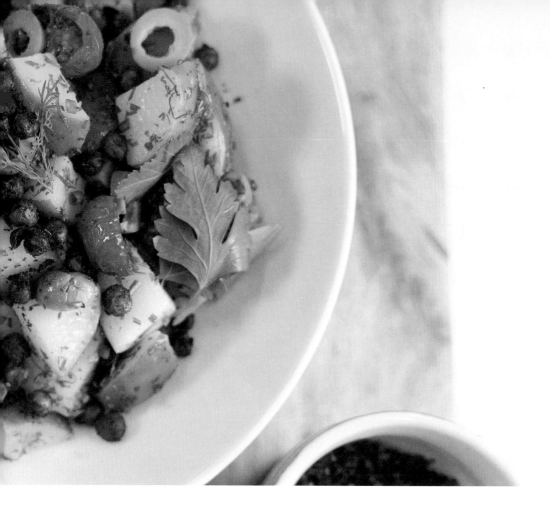

Preheat the oven to 100°C (210°F). Cut the cherry tomatoes in half, season with the olive oil, salt and pepper. Place on a baking tray and cook for about 1 hour or until semi-dried and shrivelled. Cool slightly.

In the meantime, wash and peel the potatoes and cut into 1½ cm (½ in) cubes. Heat a medium-sized pot of water and add a pinch of salt. Once simmering, add the potatoes, bring to a slow boil and cook until just done, about 5–6 minutes. Drain and spread them out to cool slightly.

In a separate bowl, combine the dressing ingredients to emulsify. Slice the olives into rondelles and place in a serving bowl with the potatoes and tomatoes. Add the herbs and spiced chickpeas, mixing well to combine. Add the dressing to taste, toss again and serve.

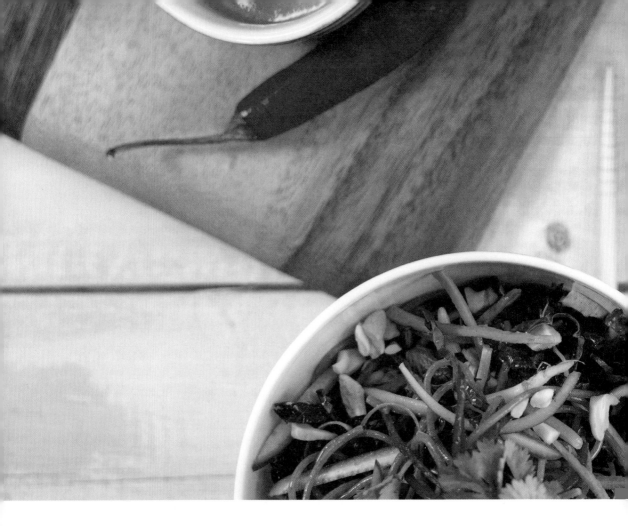

Vermicelli julienne salad with chilli, lime dressing & roasted cashews

SERVES 4

300 g (10½ oz) wholemeal vermicelli

3 Lebanese cucumbers

3 carrots

3 spring onions

200 g (7 oz) bean sprouts

4 leaves Tuscan kale

2 red chillies

1 cup coriander (cilantro) leaves, loosely packed

1 cup mint leaves, loosely packed

100 g (3½ oz) roasted cashews, finely chopped

FOR THE DRESSING

½ garlic clove, crushed

1 teaspoon fresh ginger, finely grated

20 ml (¾ fl oz) tamari or soy sauce

2 teaspoons honey

1 teaspoon lemongrass, finely chopped

80 ml (2½ fl oz) lime juice

120 ml (4 fl oz) extra virgin olive oil

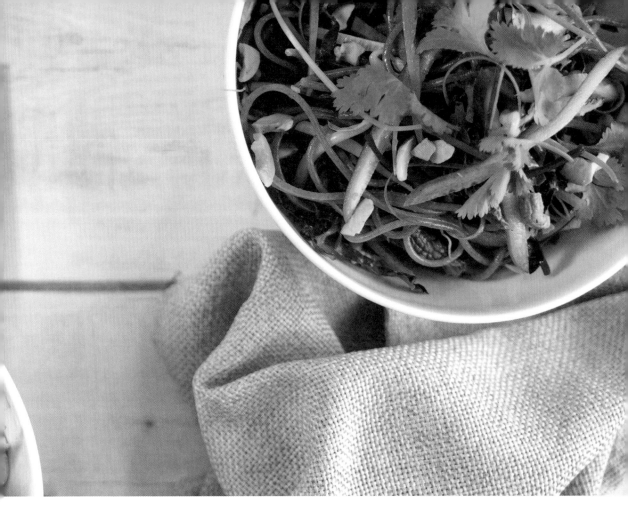

Cook the vermicelli according to the packet instructions, then drain and set aside in a bowl of cold water until needed.

Halve the cucumbers and remove the seeds. Cut into matchsticks and place in a serving bowl. Peel and julienne the carrot into fine matchsticks and add to the bowl, together with finely sliced spring onion and bean sprouts.

Remove the centre stem from the kale and finely slice each leaf. Deseed and slice the red chillies and roughly chop the coriander and mint. Add the kale, chilli, herbs and nuts to the bowl. Drain the vermicelli well and add to the serving bowl.

To make the dressing, whisk all the ingredients together in a small bowl. Drizzle the dressing over the salad. Toss well to coat. Season to taste and serve immediately.

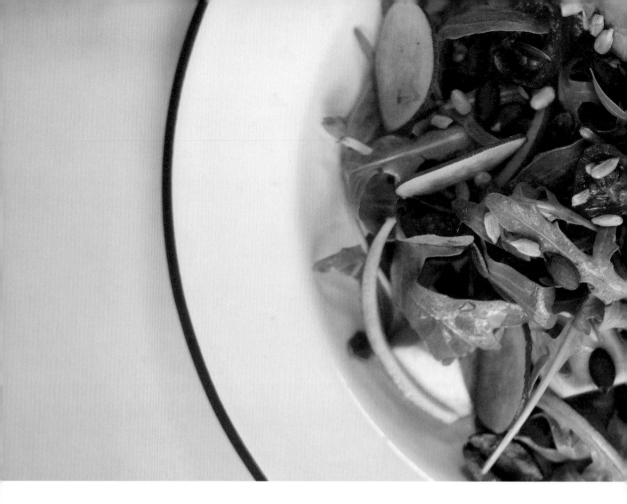

Rocket, avocado and semi-dried tomato salad with olives, seeds and balsamic dressing

SERVES 4

250 g (9 oz) cherry tomatoes

1 tablespoon extra virgin olive oil

½ tablespoon dried oregano

100 g (3½ oz) rocket (arugula)

2 avocados, diced

½ red onion, finely sliced

3 radishes, finely sliced

15 kalamata olives, pitted and halved

2 tablespoons mixed seeds (e.g., pepita, sunflower, sesame)

salt and pepper

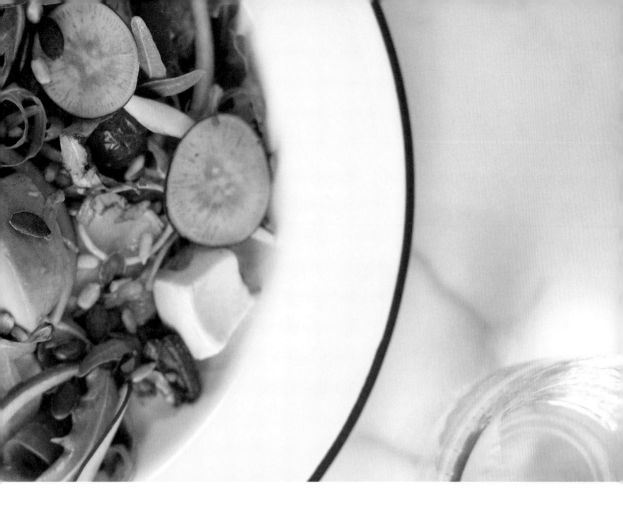

FOR THE DRESSING
60 ml (2 fl oz) balsamic vinegar

100 ml (3½ fl oz) extra virgin olive oil

1 teaspoon Dijon mustard

¼ teaspoon salt

Preheat the oven to 100°C (210°F). Cut the cherry tomatoes in half, season with the olive oil, oregano and salt and pepper. Spread on a baking tray and cook in the oven for about 1 hour, or until semi-dried and shrivelled. Cool slightly and transfer to a large serving bowl. Place all the remaining salad ingredients in the bowl and toss together.

In a separate bowl combine the dressing ingredients to emulsify. Dress the salad to taste and serve.

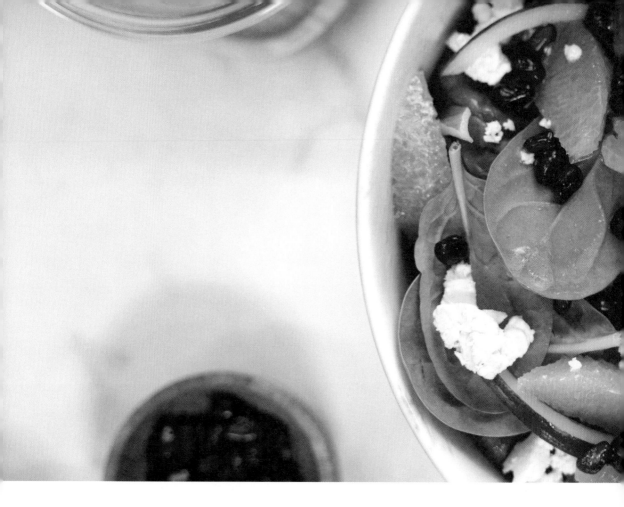

Orange, spinach and pomegranate salad with feta and brazil nuts

SERVES 4

5 oranges

½ red onion, quartered

1 large pomegranate

100 g (3½ oz) baby spinach

150 g (5½ oz) low-fat Greek feta, crumbled

¾ cup Brazil nuts, finely sliced

FOR THE DRESSING

60 ml (2 fl oz) lemon juice

120 ml (4 fl oz) extra virgin olive oil

2 teaspoons honey

¼ teaspoon salt

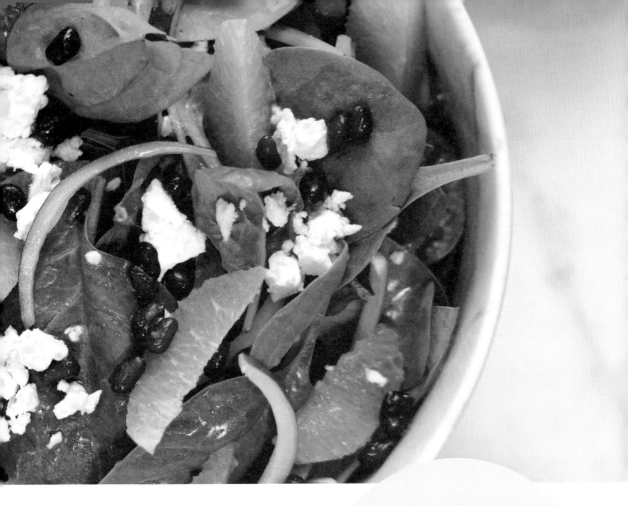

Peel the oranges and cut between the membrane to remove the flesh from each segment. Remove any seeds. Finely slice the onion and deseed the pomegranate, discarding any white parts. Place the orange segments, onion, pomegranate seeds, spinach, feta and nuts in a serving dish and mix together.

In a separate bowl combine the dressing ingredients and mix well to emulsify. Dress the salad to taste and serve.

Brazil nuts

Brazil nuts are rich in antioxidants, including selenium, vitamin E and phenols, which help combat free radicals and reduce oxidative stress. This can lower the risk of health conditions such as heart disease, diabetes, and certain cancers.

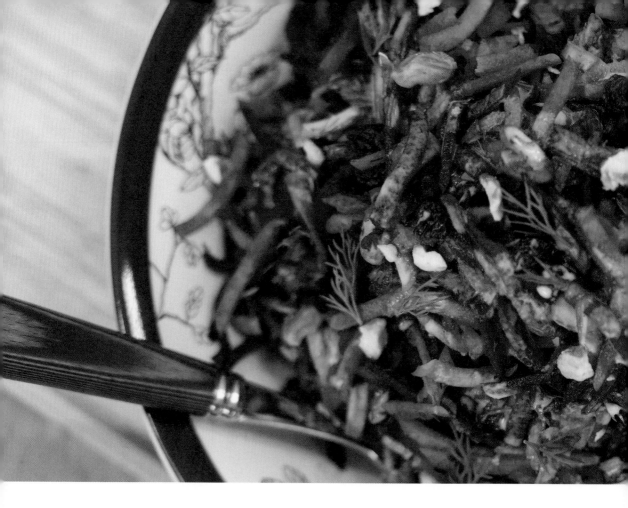

Beetroot and carrot coleslaw with sheep's yoghurt and dill

SERVES 4

3 large beetroots

3 large carrots

50 g (1¾ oz) pistachios, toasted and crushed

80 g (2¾ oz) sultanas

½ cup chopped dill, loosely packed

FOR THE DRESSING

30 ml (1 fl oz) cider vinegar

30 ml (1 fl oz) extra virgin olive oil

1 teaspoon honey

¼ teaspoon salt

100 g (3½ oz) sheep's yoghurt

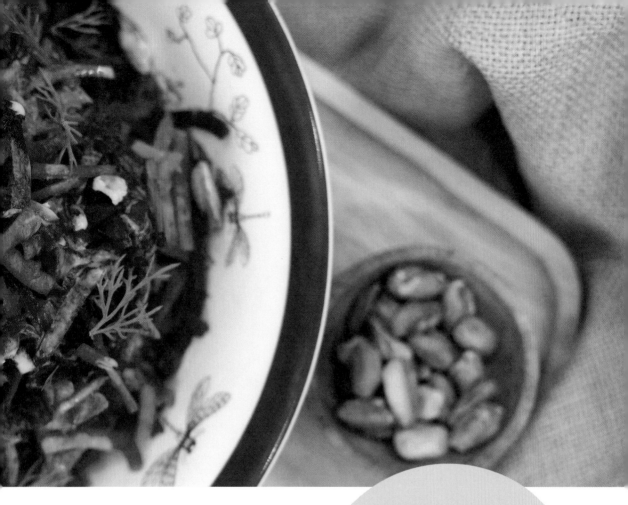

Peel and grate the beetroots and carrots. Place in a serving bowl and add the pistachios, sultanas and dill. Toss well.

In a separate bowl combine the dressing ingredients, whisking to emulsify. Dress the salad to taste and serve.

Diversity

No single food supplies all essential nutrients, so a diverse diet is key to overall wellbeing. It also keeps meals interesting and prevents monotony. To maximize the nutritional benefits of vegetables, explore options beyond your usual choices.

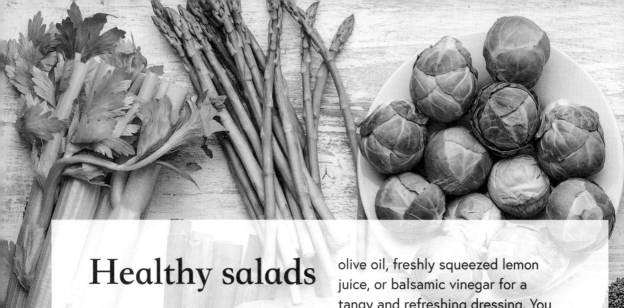

Healthy salads

There is a wide array of tender green and purple vegetables perfect for creating vibrant raw salads. These include various types of lettuce, such as loose-leaf, romaine, iceberg, and butter lettuce, as well as other leafy greens like endive, chicory, garden cress and dandelion greens.

Within the chicory family, popular varieties include radicchio and different types of endive, each bringing its own unique flavour and texture to the table.

To elevate your salad, consider adding a splash of extra-virgin olive oil, freshly squeezed lemon juice, or balsamic vinegar for a tangy and refreshing dressing. You can enhance the flavour profile by incorporating finely chopped onions or chives, which add a mild bite, or by sprinkling in nuts and seeds for a satisfying crunch. Adding ingredients like olives or capers can introduce a burst of briny richness that complements the freshness of the greens.

Experimenting with these ingredients not only creates visually appealing and colourful salads, but also ensures a nutritious, well-rounded dish that delights both the palate and the body.

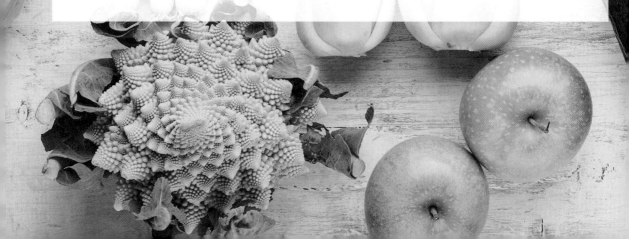

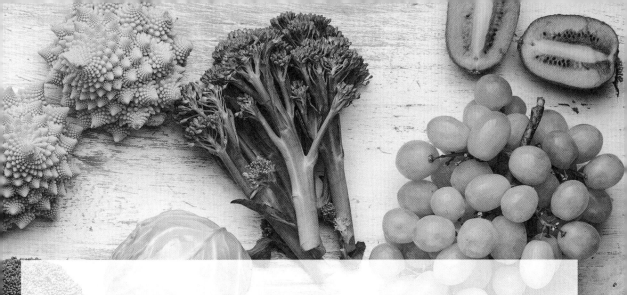

Cruciferous vegetables

Part of the family Brassicaceae, cruciferous vegetables include cabbage, broccoli, cauliflower, Brussels sprouts, kale, savoy cabbage, collard greens, watercress, rocket (arugula), bok choy, turnip greens, kohlrabi and gai lan. These interesting and healthy vegetables contain high levels of vitamin C and some unique phytochemicals, such as isothiocyanates, indol-3-carbinol and sulforophane, which seem to play a role in cancer prevention and longevity.

It is better to consume cruciferous veggies in combination with some mustard, because it contains an enzyme called myrosinase, which helps convert the dorment phytochemical glucoraphanin into the powerful cancer-suppressor molecule isothiocyanate. Add a honey mustard dressing to a slaw salad.

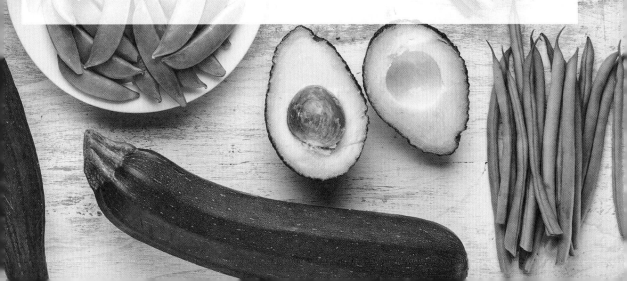

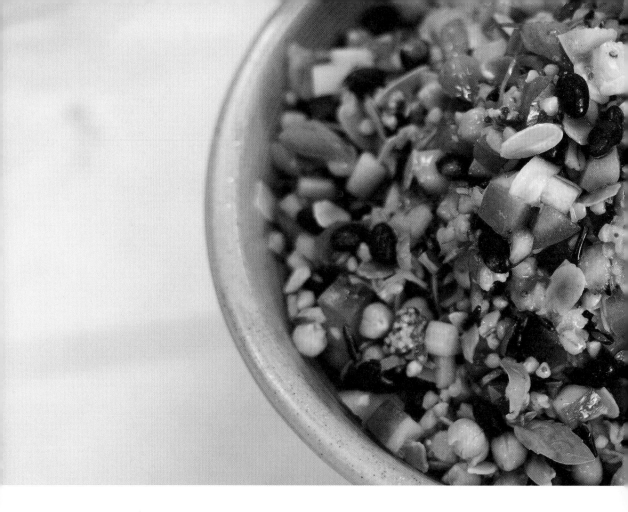

Mixed grain salad with chickpeas and black beans

SERVES 4

45 g (1½ oz) pearl barley

45 g (1½ oz) wild rice or brown rice

45 g (1½ oz) buckwheat

120 g (4½ oz) cooked chickpeas

120 g (4½ oz) cooked black beans

1 small red onion, diced

2 Lebanese cucumbers, diced

2 celery sticks, diced

2 large tomatoes, diced

70 g (2½ oz) almond flakes, toasted

2 cups basil leaves, loosely packed

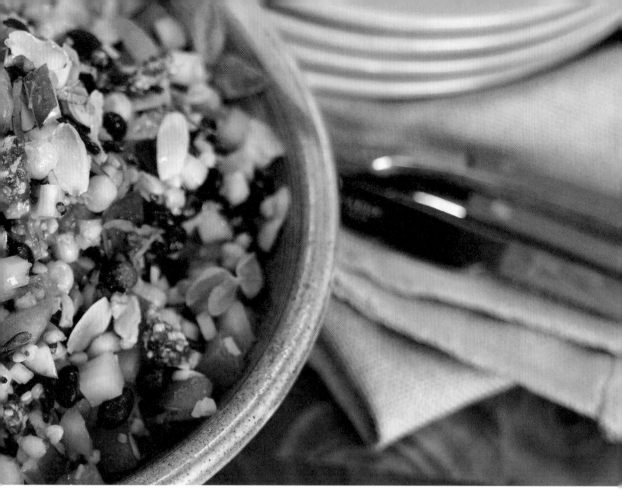

FOR THE DRESSING
60 ml (2 fl oz) lemon juice

90 ml (3 fl oz) extra virgin olive oil

20 g (¾ oz) seeded mustard

¼ teaspoon salt

½ garlic clove

35 g (1¼ oz) capers

Place a large pot of salted water on the stove and bring to a boil. Add the barley and rice. Cook for 45 minutes or until almost cooked. Add the buckwheat and cook for a further 12–15 minutes or until the buckwheat is just cooked. Drain and set aside to cool.

Prepare all the remaining salad ingredients and place in a large serving bowl. Add the grains when they are cool. Toss together well.

Place all the dressing ingredients in a blender and process until smooth. Dress the salad to taste and serve.

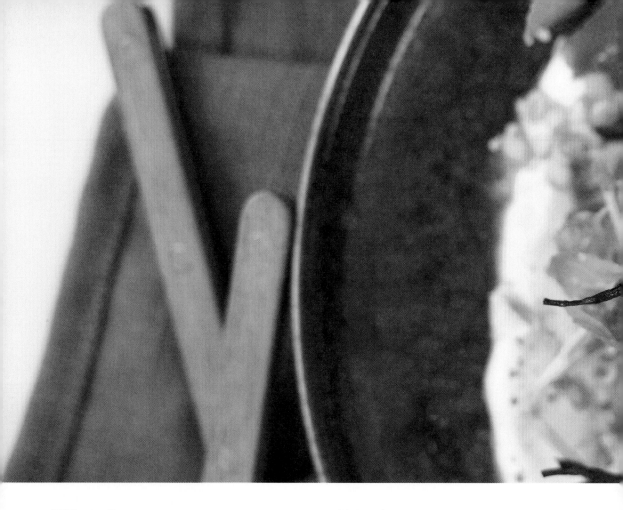

Heirloom carrots with farro, hazelnuts, sheep's yoghurt and cardamom dressing

SERVES 4

20 Dutch carrots

1 tablespoon extra virgin olive oil

100 g (3½ oz) cooked farro

4 cups watercress, loosely packed

80 g (2¾ oz) hazelnuts, roasted, peeled and slightly crushed

200 g (7 oz) sheep's yoghurt

salt and pepper

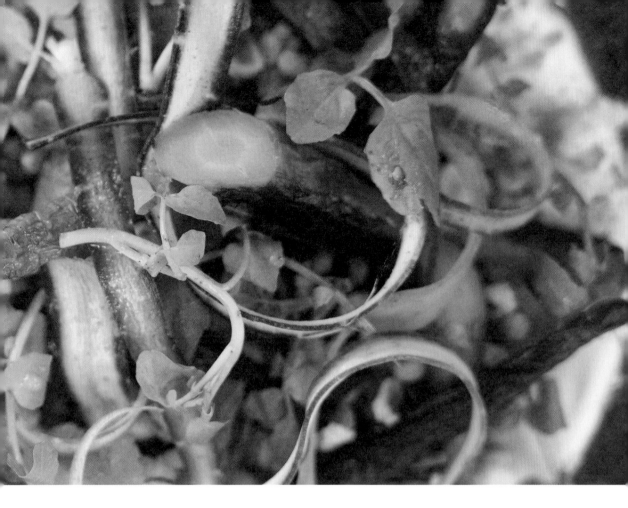

FOR THE DRESSING
60 ml (2 fl oz) extra virgin olive oil

30 ml (1 fl oz) lemon juice

30 ml (1 fl oz) orange juice

1 teaspoon orange zest

½ teaspoon ground cardamom

1 teaspoon honey

¼ teaspoon salt

Preheat the oven to 190°C (375°F). Remove the stems of the carrots and wash them well. Place 15 carrots on a baking tray and dress with the olive oil, salt and pepper. Bake until cooked through, about 25 minutes. Remove from the oven and set aside to cool. In the meantime,

Wash and pick the watercress and set aside. Using a vegetable peeler, shave the remaining raw carrots into thin strips. Once the baked carrots are cool enough to work with, cut them in half lengthways. To assemble, place all the raw and cooked carrots in a large serving bowl. Add the farro, watercress and hazelnuts and toss together well. In a separate bowl whisk the dressing ingredients until emulsified.

Spread a quarter of the yoghurt on the bottom of four plates. Dress the salad to taste and toss well. Mound the salad on top of the yoghurt and serve immediately.

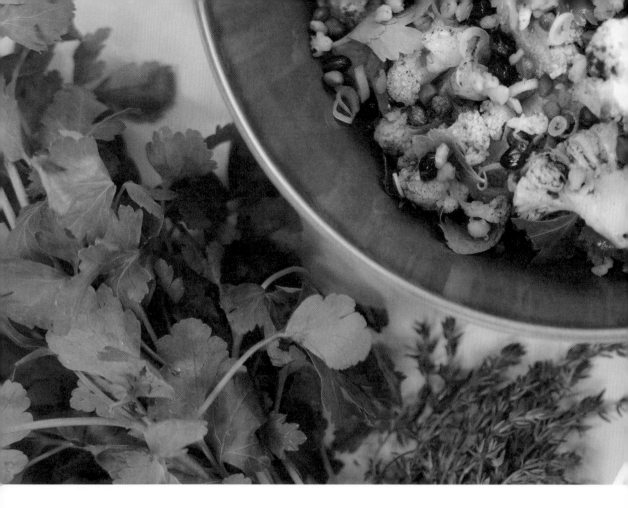

Cauliflower salad

SERVES 4

2 medium cauliflowers

1 tablespoon extra virgin olive oil

3 tablespoons capers

2 handfuls parsley leaves, roughly chopped

1 large pomegranate, deseeded

2 spring onions, finely sliced

salt and pepper to taste

FOR THE DRESSING
60 ml (2 fl oz) white wine vinegar

120 ml (4 fl oz) extra virgin olive oil

2 teaspoons seeded Dijon mustard

2 teaspoons honey

¼ teaspoon salt

1 tablespoon thyme leaves

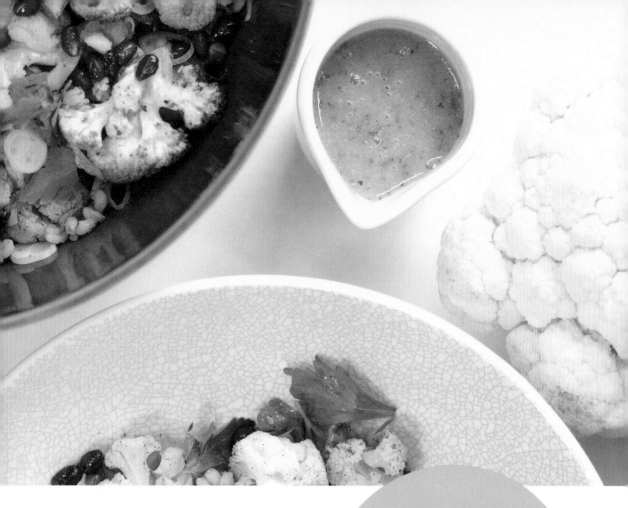

Preheat the oven to 220°C (430°F). Break down the cauliflower into florets and arrange in a single layer on a baking tray. Dress with olive oil, salt and pepper. Bake until the florets are well coloured and cooked through (15–25 minutes). Leave to cool slightly.

Place all the dressing ingredients in a bowl and whisk until combined.

Combine the cauliflower with the remaining salad ingredients in a large serving bowl. Add dressing to taste and mix well until everything is nicely coated. Check the seasoning and serve.

Parsley

Parsley is high in apigenin, a flavone that may inhibit tumour cell proliferation in cell culture studies. Other rich sources of apigenin include onions, oranges, chamomile and wheat sprouts.

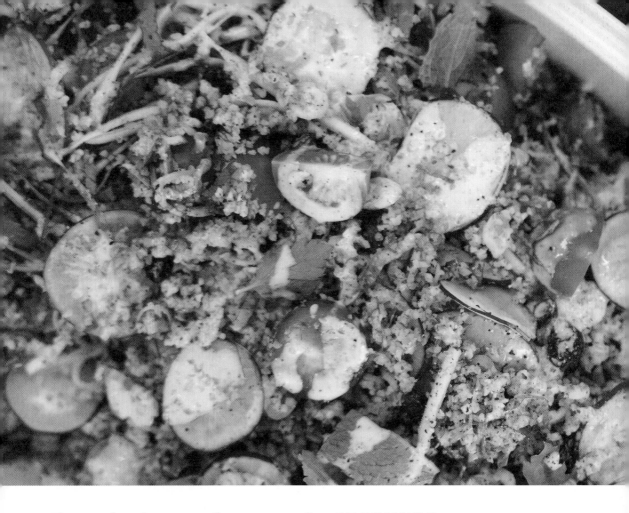

Burghul, zucchini and parsley salad with tahini dressing

SERVES 4

150 g (5½ oz) fine burghul wheat

2 large zucchini (courgette)

1½ cups flat-leaf parsley, loosely packed

1½ cups mint leaves, loosely packed

2 spring onions

6 radishes

250 g (9 oz) cherry tomatoes

75 g (2¾ oz) sultanas

FOR THE DRESSING

1 tablespoon sumac

2 teaspoons pink pepper, ground

75 ml (2½ fl oz) lemon juice

75 ml (2½ fl oz) extra virgin olive oil

1 teaspoon honey

40 g (1½ oz) tahini

40 ml (1¼ fl oz) water

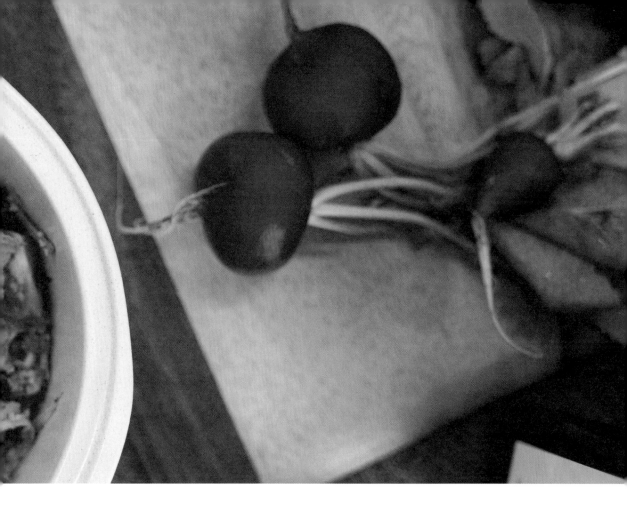

Place the burghul in a medium-sized heatproof bowl. Boil 300 ml (10 fl oz) of water and pour over the burghul. Cover and set aside for 20 minutes to soften. Drain any excess liquid off.

Coarsely grate the zucchini and place in a large serving bowl. Using your hands, roughly tear the parsley and mint and add to the bowl. Finely slice the spring onions and radishes and quarter the cherry tomatoes. Combine them in the bowl along with the sultanas and cooked burghul. Mix well.

In a separate bowl combine the dressing ingredients to emulsify. Dress the salad to taste, mix well and serve.

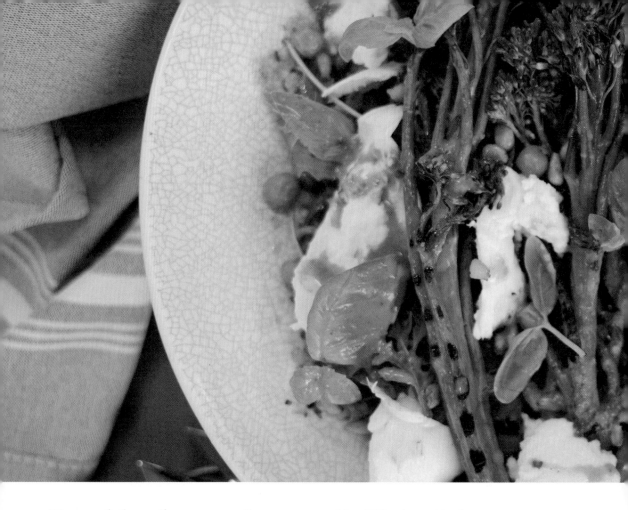

Pearl barley, rocket, grilled broccolini and mozzarella salad with basil dressing

SERVES 4

80 g (2¾ oz) pearl barley

250 g (9 oz) frozen peas

2 bunches broccolini

1 tablespoon extra virgin olive oil

60 g (2 oz) rocket (arugula)

80 g (2¾ oz) pine nuts, toasted

1 buffalo mozzarella ball, torn into pieces

½ cup basil leaves

salt and pepper to taste

FOR THE DRESSING

60 ml (2 fl oz) lemon juice

120 ml (4 fl oz) extra virgin olive oil

¼ teaspoon salt

1 cup basil leaves, loosely packed

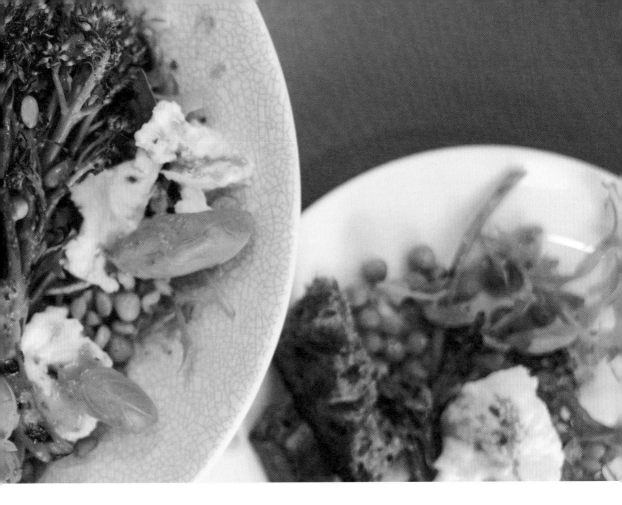

Place a medium saucepan of water over high heat with a pinch of salt. Bring to the boil and add the pearl barley. Cook until almost done (about 45–55 minutes), then add the peas and cook for a further 1–2 minutes. Drain and set aside to cool.

Trim the broccolini of any woody ends or extra leaves. Place in a bowl and season with the olive oil. salt and pepper. Cook the broccolini on a hot grill or grill pan making sure the stems are cooked through and the tops are not burnt.

In the meantime, place all the dressing ingredients in a blender and process until smooth.

Combine the barley, peas, broccolini and rocket in a large serving bowl. Dress to taste, tossing well. Serve topped with the pine nuts, mozzarella and basil.

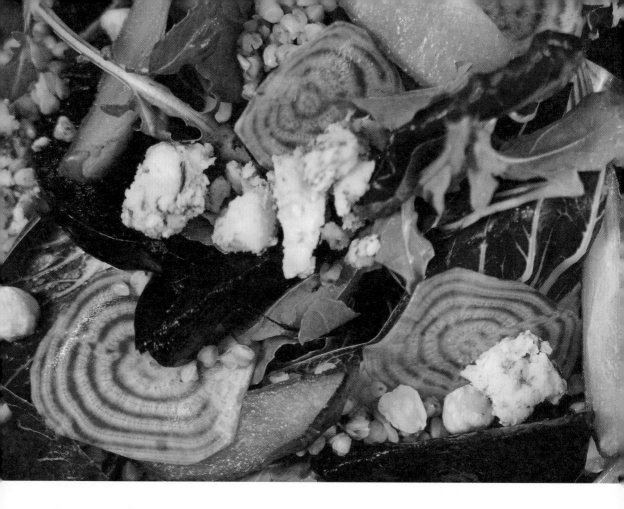

Bitter leaves and beetroot salad with pear, hazelnut and blue cheese

SERVES 4

4 large beetroots, washed

4 firm pears

1 tablespoon honey

½ teaspoon ground cinnamon

150 g (5½ oz) buckwheat

200 g (7 oz) rocket (arugula)

2 small radicchio, washed and sliced

150 g (5½ oz) Stilton cheese, crumbled

40 g (1½ oz) hazelnuts, roasted, peeled and crushed

FOR THE DRESSING

40 g (1½ oz) hazelnut butter

40 ml (1¼ fl oz) pomegranate molasses

30 ml (1 fl oz) balsamic vinegar

¼ teaspoon salt

65 ml (2¼ fl oz) water

freshly ground pepper to taste

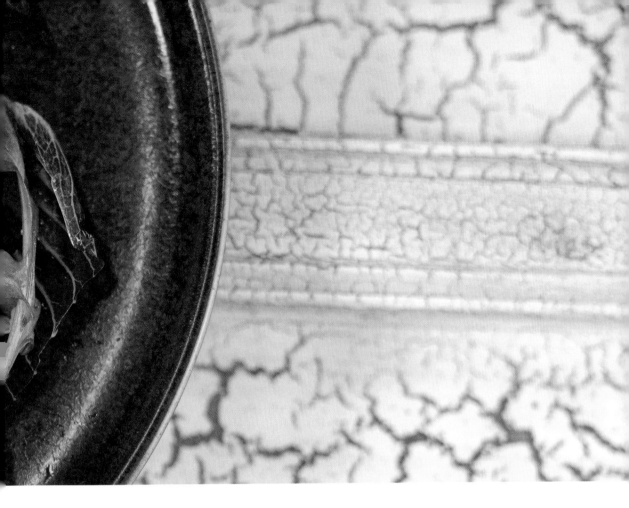

Preheat the oven to 200°C (400°F). Wrap the beetroots separately in aluminium foil and place on a baking sheet in the oven. Cook until a knife can easily pierce the flesh (about 1 hour). Set aside to cool.

In the meantime, quarter the pears, remove the core and cut into thin wedges. Place the pears in a bowl and coat evenly with the honey and cinnamon. Arrange on a lined baking tray. Once the beetroots are cooked, lower the temperature of the oven to 180°C (350°F) and transfer the tray of pears. Bake for 15–20 minutes, until cooked through and slightly caramelised. Set aside to cool slightly.

Meanwhile, cook the buckwheat in plenty of salted boiling water for about 12 minutes or until tender. Drain and set aside. For the dressing, place all the ingredients in a bowl and whisk until combined.

When the beetroots are cool enough to handle, peel them and cut into bite-sized wedges. Place the pears, buckwheat, rocket and radicchio into a serving dish and toss well. Add the beetroot, cheese and nuts. Mix again, then serve, drizzled with the dressing as desired.

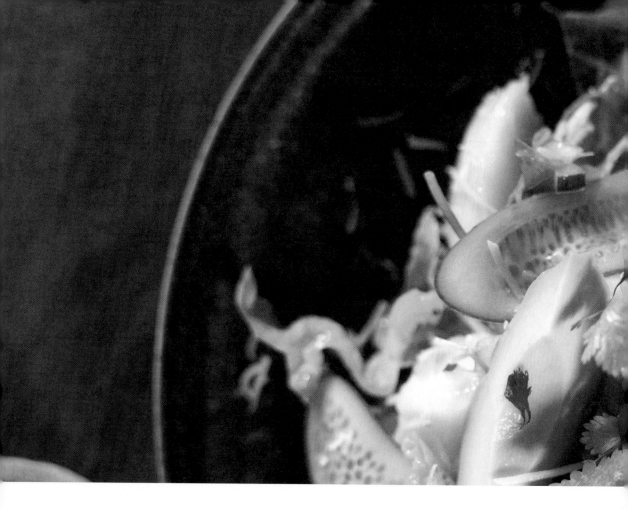

Avocado and mango salad with makrut lime dressing

SERVES 4

40 g (1½ oz) shredded coconut

2 ripe mangos

2 ripe avocados

4 Lebanese cucumbers

2 baby gem lettuces

½ red onion, finely diced

2 handfuls coriander (cilantro) leaves, picked

2 medium red chillies, deseeded and sliced

FOR THE DRESSING

1 or 2 makrut lime leaves

zest of 1 lime

60 ml (2 fl oz) lime juice

120 ml (4 fl oz) extra virgin olive oil

2 teaspoons honey

¼ teaspoon salt

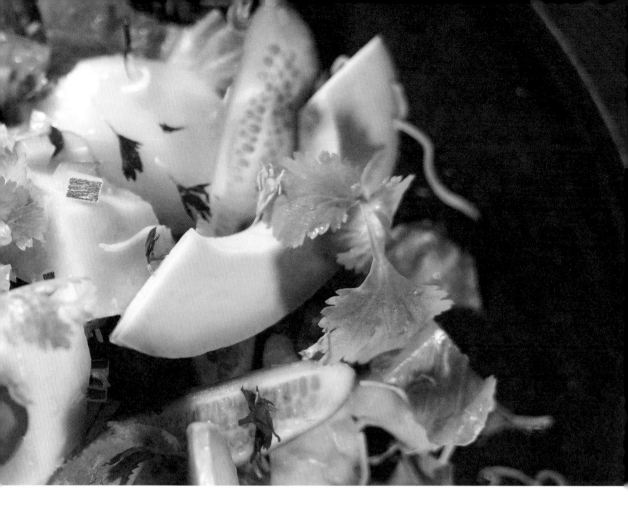

Preheat the oven to 160°C (320°F). Place the coconut on a baking tray and cook until lightly browned, about 5–10 minutes. Set aside to cool. In the meantime, cut the mango and avocado into 2½ cm (1 in) dice. Using a vegetable peeler, shave the cucumbers lengthways, stopping when you get to the seeds. Rotate the cucumbers and shave until all sides are done and you are left with long curls of seedless flesh. Wash the lettuce well and cut into 2½ cm (1 in) slices.

To prepare the dressing, remove the central vein of the lime leaves and discard it. With a sharp knife chop the leaves into very thin slices. Collect them together and slice again in the opposite direction. Keep chopping until it is very finely diced. Place in a small bowl and add all the remaining dressing ingredients. Whisk until combined.

Gently combine all the salad ingredients in a salad bowl or serving plate. Serve with the dressing.

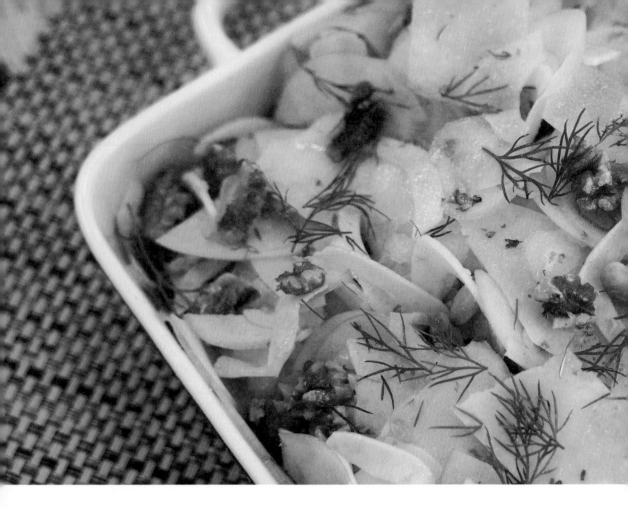

Apple and fennel salad with pecorino and walnuts

SERVES 4

200 g (7 oz) frozen edamame

1 medium fennel bulb

2 granny smith apples

3 celery sticks

80 g (2¾ oz) toasted walnuts, chopped

½ bunch dill, picked and finely chopped

35 g (1¼ oz) pecorino cheese, shaved

FOR THE DRESSING

60 ml (2 fl oz) lime juice

120 ml (4 fl oz) extra virgin olive oil

2 teaspoons honey

¼ teaspoon salt

1 tablespoon wasabi

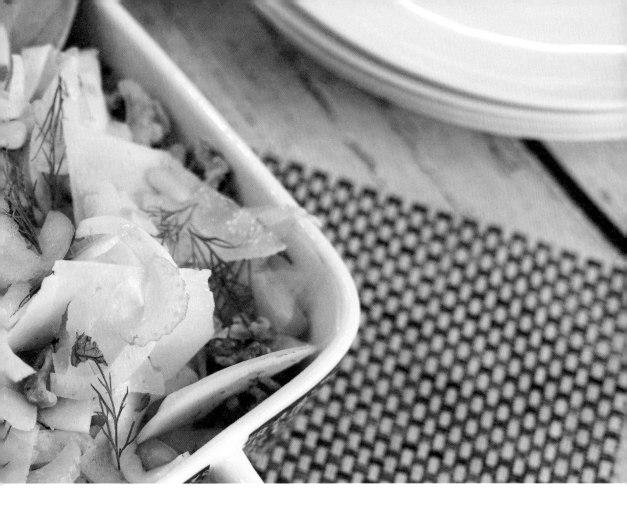

Bring a medium saucepan of salted water to a boil. Add the edamame and cook for 2 minutes. Strain and set aside to cool.

Trim the fennel bulb and cut it in half. Cut the cheeks off the apples and discard the cores. Thinly slice the fennel, apple and celery using a mandoline or cut by hand. Combine all the salad ingredients in a serving bowl and toss well.

Place all the dressing ingredients in a small bowl and whisk to emulsify. Dress the salad to taste and serve.

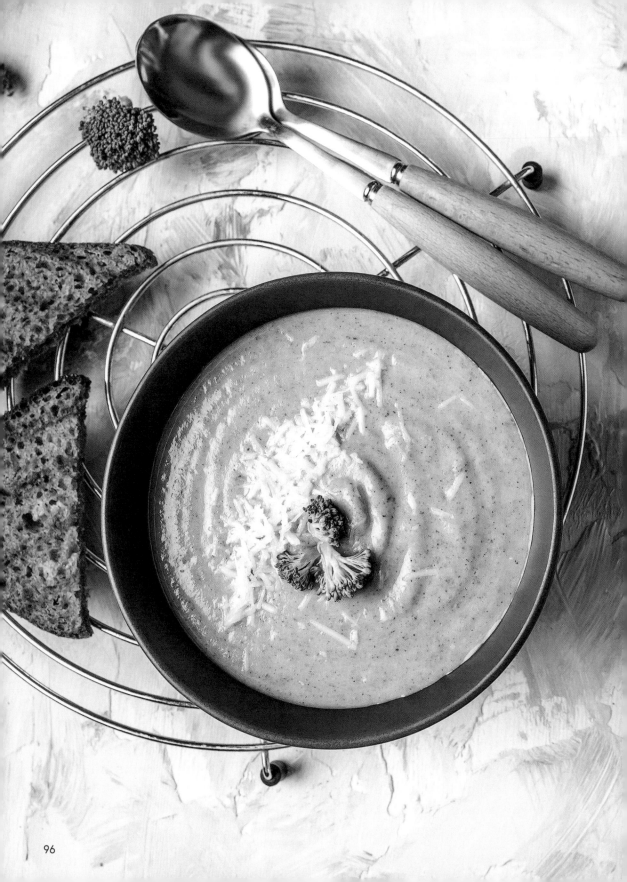

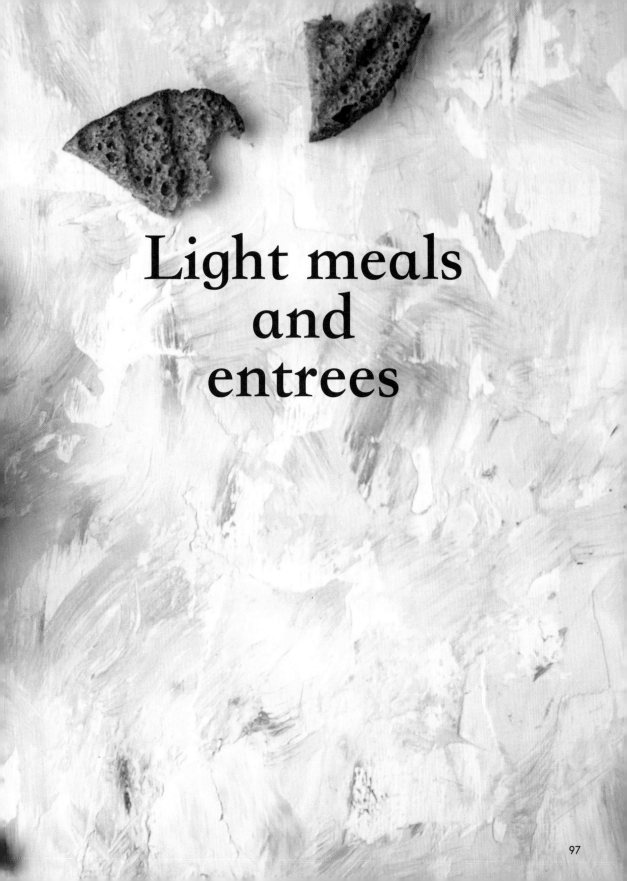

Light meals and entrees

Ethiopian hummus with wholemeal grissini

SERVES 4

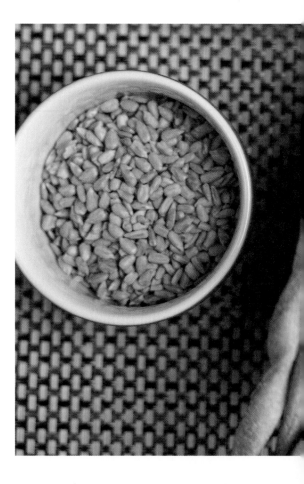

FOR THE GRISSINI

280 g (10 oz) wholemeal flour

7 g (¼ oz) salt

4 g (⅛ oz) baker's yeast

190 ml (6½ fl oz) warm water

1 teaspoon honey

1 tablespoon extra virgin olive oil

FOR THE HUMMUS

450 g (1 lb) drained cooked chickpeas
  (keep ¾ cup cooking or can liquid)

80 g (2¾ oz) raw sunflower seeds

2 garlic cloves, finely sliced

60 ml (2 fl oz) lemon juice

1 green chilli, deseeded

40 ml (1½ fl oz) extra virgin olive oil

½ teaspoon ground cardamom

1 teaspoon smoked paprika

½ teaspoon ground coriander

½ teaspoon ground fenugreek

¼ teaspoon ground nutmeg

¼ teaspoon ground clove

salt and pepper to taste

Place the flour and salt in the bowl of a stand mixer. In a separate bowl mix the yeast, water, honey and oil. Start the mixer on a low setting with the hook attachment. Slowly pour in the liquid yeast mixture and keep mixing until a velvety dough is formed. Cover with cling wrap and refrigerate for 2–12 hours.

When ready, preheat the oven to 190°C (375 °F). Transfer the dough to a lightly floured bench and roll using a rolling pin to ½ cm (¼ in) thickness. Cut the dough into 1 cm (½ in) strips and, holding the two ends with your fingers, twist the strips to form a spiral. Transfer to a lined baking tray and cook until golden brown and crisp, about 20–25 minutes. If the grissini are golden but not crisp all the way through, reduce

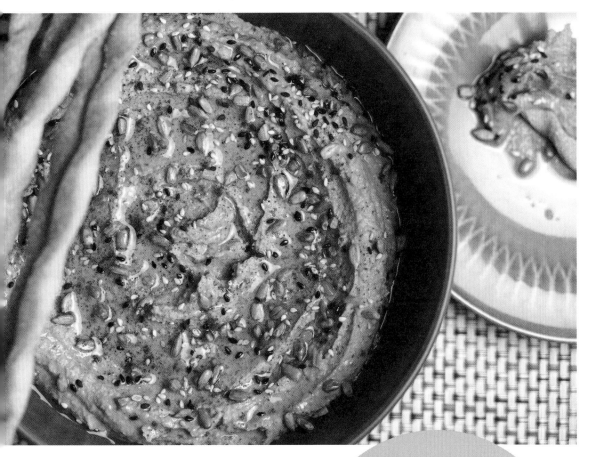

the temperature to 120°C (250°F) and return the grissini to bake for a few more minutes. Remove to a rack to cool.

Place all the hummus ingredients in a food processor and blend until very smooth. Adjust the salt to taste, transfer to a serving bowl and serve with the grissini.

Chickpeas

A concentrated source of protein, dietary fibre, vitamins, minerals and low-glycaemic starches – one cup of boiled chickpeas contains 270 calories, 12 g of dietary fibre, 15 g of protein and 4 g of fat (mainly mono- and poly-unsaturated). Chickpeas also provide plenty of folate which is essential for our health.

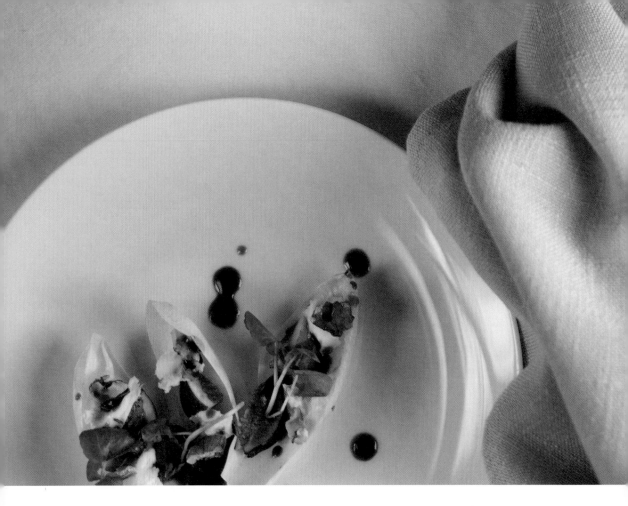

Endive cups with blue cheese, walnuts, figs and rosemary balsamic vinegar dressing

SERVES 4

FOR THE DRESSING

120 ml (4 fl oz) balsamic vinegar

2 teaspoons honey

1 sprig of rosemary, roughly chopped

⅛ teaspoon freshly ground pepper

30 ml (1 fl oz) extra virgin olive oil

FOR THE CUPS

3 endives

½ bunch watercress

300 g (10½ oz) ripe figs

120 g (4½ oz) Gorgonzola dolce, crumbled

80 g (2¾ oz) toasted walnuts, chopped

salt and pepper to taste

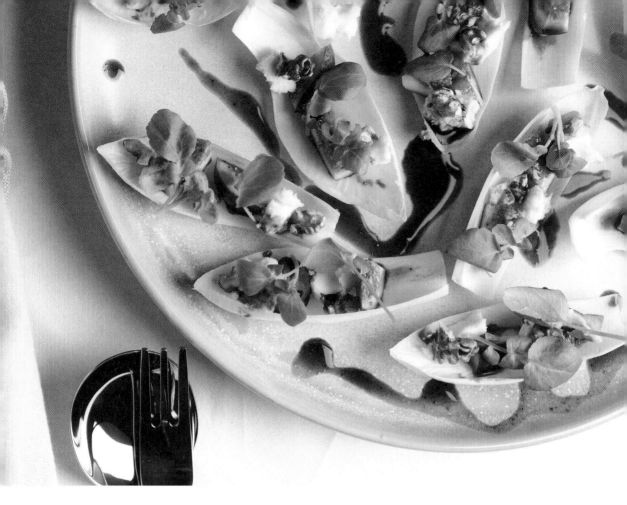

For the dressing, place the vinegar, honey, rosemary and pepper in a small saucepan and bring to a simmer. Keep simmering until it has reduced by half, no more. Set aside to cool. Once cool, strain. Just before serving, vigorously whisk in the olive oil.

In the meantime, cut the base off the endives. Separate the leaves, wash and dry them. Arrange the leaves, facing up like cups, on a serving platter. Wash and dry the watercress and pick the nicest sprigs. Set aside. Cut the figs into wedges.

Evenly divide the figs, cheese and walnuts in the endive cups. Top with sprigs of watercress, dress with the balsamic reduction and season with salt and pepper..

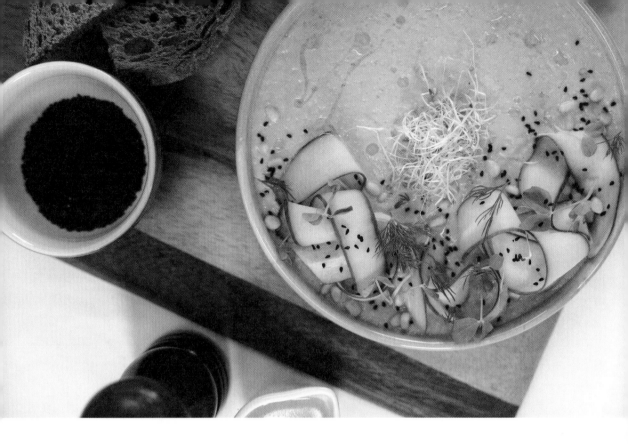

Cucumber, pea and avocado gazpacho

SERVES 4

FOR THE SOUP

350 g (12½ oz) sliced cucumber

70 g (2½ oz) frozen peas

1 medium avocado

¼ red onion

2 long green chillis, deseeded

1 garlic clove

1 cup coriander (cilantro) leaves, loosely packed

1 cup mint leaves, loosely packed

300 ml (10 fl oz) rice milk

60 ml (2 fl oz) lime juice

2 tablespoons extra virgin olive oil

salt and pepper to taste

TO SERVE

1 Lebanese cucumber, thinly shaved

1 cup alfalfa sprouts

½ cup dill leaves, finely chopped

30 g (1 oz) pine nuts, toasted

1 tablespoon nigella seeds

Place all the ingredients for the gazpacho in a high-speed blender and liquidise well. Serve chilled or at room temperature, topped with the green garnishes, pine nuts and nigella.

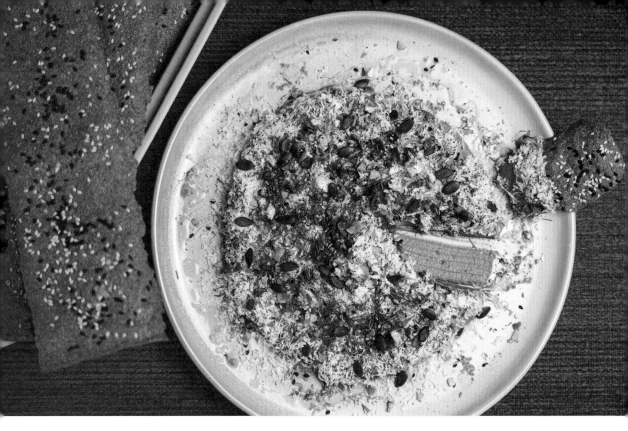

Spinach & tofu dip

SERVES 4

100 g (3½ oz) raw cashews

1 small onion, finely chopped

4 garlic cloves, sliced

½ tablespoon extra virgin olive oil

200 g (7 oz) medium-firm tofu

1½ teaspoons nutritional yeast

350 g (12½ oz) blanched and squeezed
spinach (or defrosted and well-squeezed
frozen spinach)

35 ml (1¼ fl oz) lemon juice

⅛ teaspoon ground nutmeg

salt and pepper to taste

1 tablespoon chopped dill

20 g (¾ oz) grated parmesan

1 tablespoon roasted pepitas

½ tablespoon dukkah

Lavosh (page 184)

Soak the cashews in hot water for 2 hours. In
the meantime, using a frying pan over a medium
heat, slowly sweat the onion and garlic in the
olive oil until translucent. Set aside until cool.

Drain the cashews well and transfer to a high-
speed blender with the sweated onion and
garlic, tofu and nutritional yeast. Blend until
smooth. Add the squeezed spinach, lemon juice
and nutmeg. Blend again and season with salt
and pepper to taste.

Transfer the dip to a serving bowl and top with
the dill, parmesan, pepitas and dukkah. Serve
with lavosh.

Eggplant and tomato with buckwheat crispbread

SERVES 4

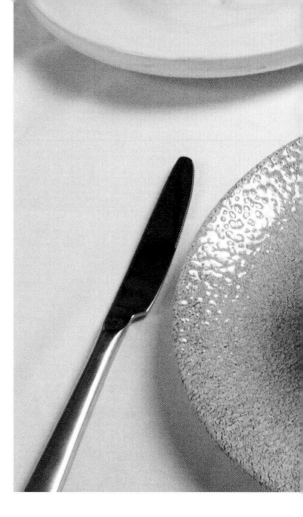

FOR THE EGGPLANT LAYER
3 medium eggplants (aubergine)

1 French eschalot

½ garlic clove

1½ tablespoons natural yoghurt

1½ teaspoons fresh oregano, chopped

½ teaspoon lemon juice

½ teaspoon lemon zest

¼ teaspoon ground cumin

¼ teaspoon ground coriander

1½ teaspoons extra virgin olive oil

1 teaspoon tahini

salt and cracked black pepper to taste

FOR THE TOMATO LAYER
10 tomatoes

1 tablespoon basil leaves, sliced

1 tablespoon white balsamic vinegar

½ tablespoon extra virgin olive oil

FOR THE GARNISH
1 small radicchio

½ bunch watercress

1 handful rocket (arugula) leaves

1 tablespoon extra virgin olive oil

1 tablespoon lemon juice

salt and pepper to taste

Buckwheat crispbread (page 177)

For the eggplant, prick the eggplants a few times with a skewer and place on a live flame over a gas jet or on a BBQ. At the same time, bring a large pot of water to the boil. Char the eggplant very well on each side (about 5–7 minutes each side) and keep turning until the whole eggplant is completely blistered and the inside cooked. In the meantime, finely dice the French eschalot and mince the garlic. Set aside.

Once the eggplants are cooked, using a paring knife, peel off the skin while leaving the flesh intact. Press the flesh between two trays and refrigerate for 3–4 hours. Try to end up with a 1 cm (½ in) slab of eggplant.

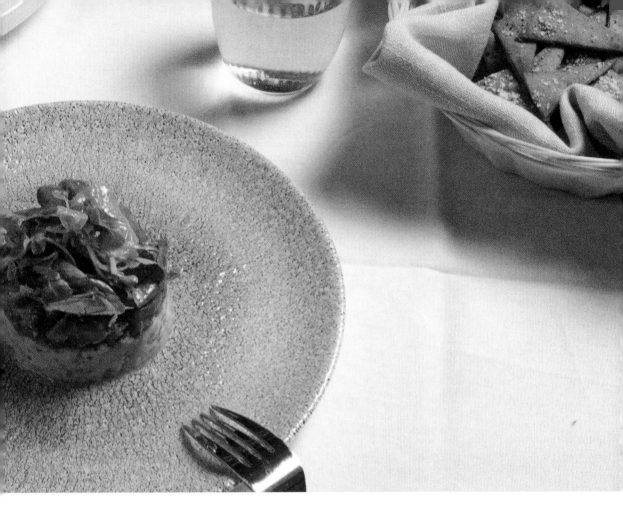

In the meantime, for the tomato layer, remove the sepal of each tomato using a sharp knife and score an x mark on the bottom of each. Blanch the tomatoes in boiling water and refresh in ice water for just long enough to peel the skin (30–60 seconds). Discard the skin. Quarter the tomatoes and remove the seeds, leaving only the seedless, skinless flesh. Dice in 1 cm (½ in) pieces and place in a small bowl. Dress and add the basil leaves just before assembling.

Once the eggplant is cold and set, discard any liquid and cut the flesh into 1 cm (½ in) cubes. Place the eggplant in a small bowl and dress with all the remaining ingredients including the reserved eschalot and garlic.

To prepare the garnish, cut the radicchio into 2½ cm (1 in) pieces, wash and pick the watercress and rocket. Combine in a bowl and dress with the olive oil, lemon, salt and pepper.

When ready to serve, use a ring mould to create the tartare layers. Spoon and press down each of the layers and top with the radicchio garnish. Serve with Buckwheat crispbread.

Wholemeal panzarotti with eggplant, cherry tomato and basil

SERVES 6

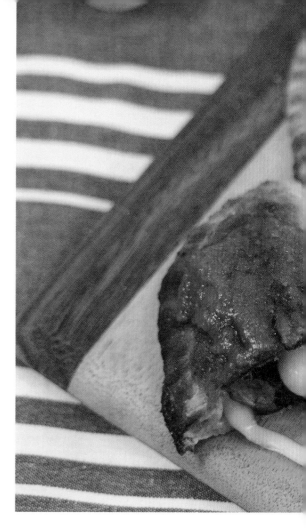

FOR THE DOUGH

450 g (1 lb) wholemeal strong flour

10 g (¼ oz) salt

330 ml (10 fl oz) warm water

¼ teaspoon baker's yeast

100 g (3½ oz) sourdough starter (50% hydration) or additional ¼ teaspoon baker's yeast

20 ml (¾ fl oz) extra virgin olive oil

1 teaspoon honey

2 medium eggplants

4 tablespoons extra virgin olive oil

200 g (7 oz) cherry tomatoes

1 tablespoon dried oregano

200 g (7 oz) tomato sugo (page 140)

350 g (12½ oz) mozzarella, grated

1 cup basil leaves, loosely packed

50 g (1¾ oz) grated parmesan

salt and pepper to taste

To make the dough, ideally start the day before. Place the flour and salt in a large bowl. Mix well and form a well in the middle. In a separate bowl, combine the water, yeast, sourdough starter, oil and honey. Mix thoroughly and allow to sit for 2 minutes. Pour the liquids into the flour, slowly incorporating the mix, working from the outside to the centre using a wooden spoon or your hands. Keep mixing until a dough

has formed. Transfer the dough onto a lightly floured bench and knead for 2–3 minutes or until the dough is stretchy and smooth. Wipe the bowl of any residue and brush the inside lightly with olive oil. Place the dough back in the bowl, cover with cling wrap and refrigerate overnight (or from 6–24 hours).

The next day, portion the dough into 12 balls, rolling and shaping them gently with your hands. Place the balls on a lightly floured tray and cover with a damp cloth. Place in a warm area until the dough has doubled in size. Once the dough has risen, transfer to a lightly floured surface and stretch into circles ½ cm (¼ in) thick.

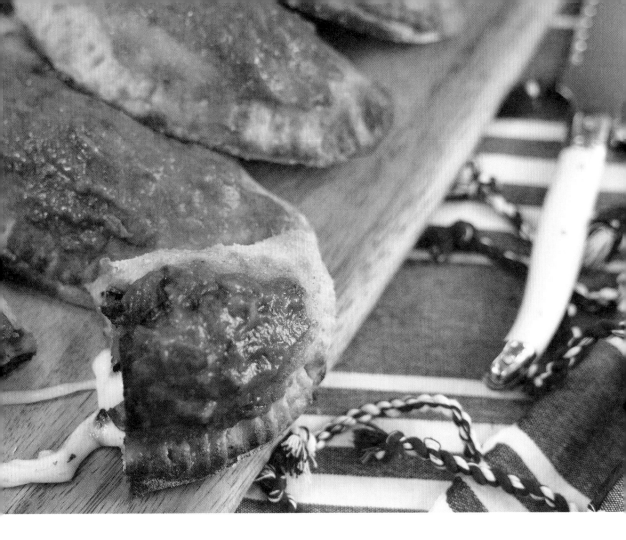

In the meantime, preheat the oven to 240°C (460°F). Cut the eggplant into 2½ cm (1 in) cubes and place in a bowl. Toss with 3 tablespoons of olive oil and season with salt and pepper to taste. Place the eggplant on a lined baking sheet and roast for 20 minutes, turning the pieces halfway through the cooking time. Remove when cooked through and well coloured. Cut the cherry tomatoes in half and season with the oregano and salt and pepper. Set aside.

To assemble, spread a tablespoon of sugo on one half of each circle, leaving 1 cm (½ in) clean edge around the outside of the dough, and place the mozzarella, eggplant, cherry tomatoes and basil on top. Fold the dough over the filled half to make a crescent shape and seal the edges by pressing down with the back of a fork.

Transfer the panzarotti to a lined baking tray and brush the tops lightly with olive oil. Bake until the panzarotti puff up and the dough takes on a rich golden colour, about 10–15 minutes. Top with a little extra sugo and parmesan to serve.

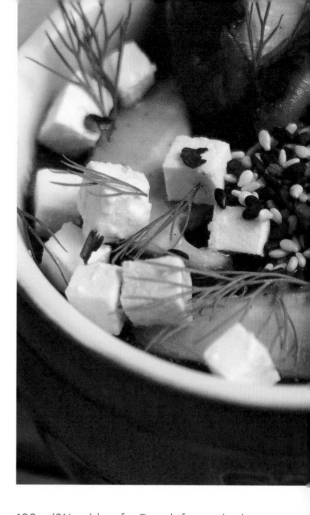

Set spinach custard with pickled mushrooms, feta and sesame

SERVES 4

FOR THE PICKLED MUSHROOMS

250 g (9 oz) shimeji mushrooms

150 ml (5 fl oz) rice vinegar

1 tablespoon honey

½ teaspoon salt

FOR THE CUSTARD

600 g (1lb 5 oz) fresh spinach or 290 g (10 oz) frozen spinach

250 ml (8½ fl oz) vegetable stock

3 large eggs

⅛ teaspoon ground nutmeg

salt and pepper to taste

100 g (3½ oz) low-fat Danish feta, cubed or crumbled

1 tablespoon white sesame seeds

1 tablespoon black sesame seeds

¼ cup dill leaves, chopped

chilli flakes

Using a paring knife, separate the shimeji mushrooms into single stems. In a medium saucepan over a high heat bring 350 ml (12 fl oz) water to the boil with the vinegar, honey and salt. Add the mushrooms and bring back to a boil. Remove pan from the heat, leaving the mushrooms in the liquid until needed.

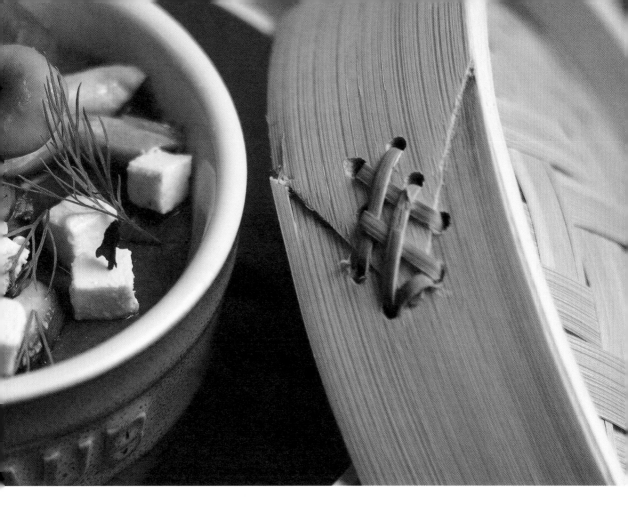

If you are using fresh spinach, fill another large pot with water, add a big pinch of salt and bring to the boil. Blanch the spinach in the boiling water, remove to a colander and set aside to cool. Squeeze out as much water as possible. If using frozen spinach, the blanching step is not needed, only thawing and squeezing. Whichever spinach you use, make sure there is enough to make 250 g (9 oz) final weight after squeezing.

Place the spinach and remaining custard ingredients in a blender and liquidise thoroughly.

Pour the liquid through a fine strainer into a bowl or jug. Discard the solids. Divide the custard between four small heatproof ramekins or bowls. Cover tightly with microwave-safe plastic wrap. Bring 2½ cm (1 in) of water to a simmer in a pan fitted with a steamer basket and lid. Add ramekins to the steamer. Cover the steamer and gently boil over a medium-low heat until the custard has set, about 15 minutes. Unwrap the custards and serve with the mushrooms, feta, sesame, dill and chilli flakes.

Seitan tandoori skewers with herbed yoghurt

SERVES 4

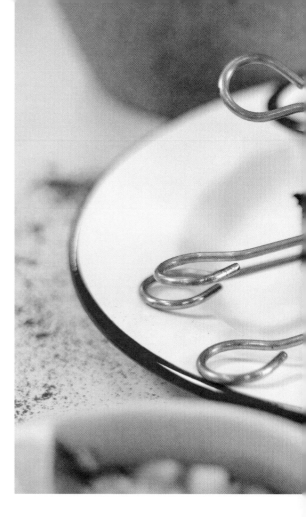

FOR THE SEITAN

320 g (11½ oz) vital wheat gluten

2 tablespoons besan flour

2 tablespoons nutritional yeast

½ teaspoon baking soda

2 teaspoons onion powder

260 ml (9 fl oz) vegetable stock plus 2 litres
  (68 fl oz) for poaching

30 g (1 oz) soy sauce

40 g (1½ oz) tomato paste

30 g (1 oz) extra virgin olive oil

FOR THE TANDOORI PASTE

200 g (7 oz) low-fat natural yoghurt

2 teaspoons turmeric

3 teaspoons ground coriander

2 teaspoons garam masala

1 teaspoon ground fennel seed

¼ teaspoon chilli powder

¼ teaspoon ground black pepper

6 teaspoons paprika

2 teaspoons garlic powder

2 teaspoons ground ginger

2 teaspoons fenugreek, ground

20 g (¾ oz) extra virgin olive oil

salt to taste

FOR THE YOGHURT

200 g (7 oz) low-fat natural yoghurt

1 small green chilli, deseeded

¼ cup mint leaves, chopped

¼ cup coriander (cilantro) leaves, chopped

20 ml (¾ fl oz) lemon juice

1 small cucumber, seeds removed

salt and pepper to taste

The day before, make and poach the seitan. Combine the vital wheat gluten, besan flour, yeast, baking soda and onion powder in a mixing bowl. Add the remaining seitan ingredients and mix using a wooden spoon until a dough is formed.

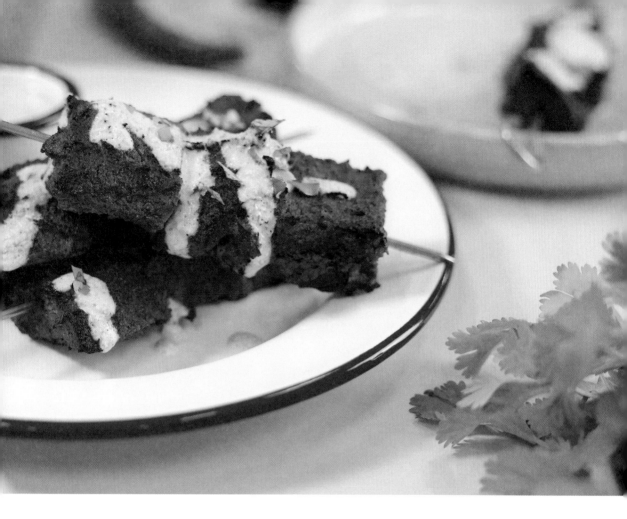

Knead the dough until well combined and form into a disk.

In a large saucepan, bring the remaining vegetable stock to a gentle simmer. Add the dough and cook for 15–20 minutes never allowing the liquid to come to a full rolling boil.

Remove the poached seitan and place on a baking sheet, with another baking sheet weighted on top. Place in the fridge to set overnight.

The next day, preheat the oven to 220°C (430°F). Meanwhile, make the tandoori paste by combining all the ingredients in a bowl and mixing well until fully incorporated. For the yoghurt, place all the ingredients in a blender and blitz until smooth. Chill in the fridge until ready.

Cut the chilled seitan into 2½ cm (1 in) cubes and place in a bowl. Add the tandoori paste and mix thoroughly until all the cubes are well coated. Thread the cubes onto skewers and place onto a lined baking tray. Bake until well coloured, about 10–15 minutes, and serve with the herbed yoghurt.

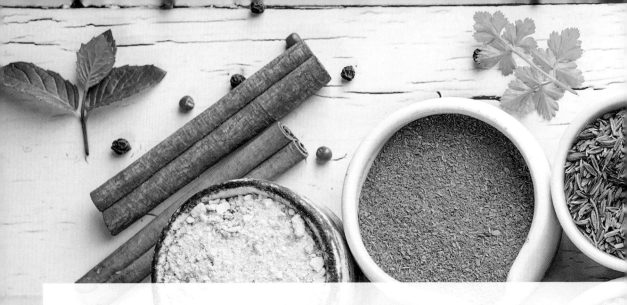

Herbs and spices

Since antiquity, culinary herbs and spices have been used to provide a wonderful range of flavours, aromas and colour to our food, as well as being used as preservatives because of their antimicrobial and antiviral properties.

Another reason to incorporate flavourful fresh, dried or powdered herbs and spices in your recipes is to reduce the consumption of less healthy ingredients such as salt, sugar, butter and vegetable oils. Chilli pepper, basil, parsley, coriander (cilantro), dill, rosemary, sage, thyme, oregano, turmeric, black pepper, cumin, caraway and many other herbal seasonings can transform a so-so recipe into a memorable

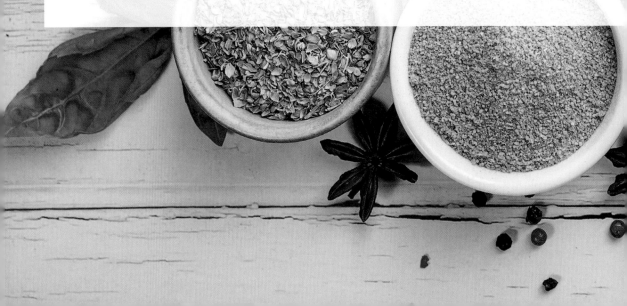

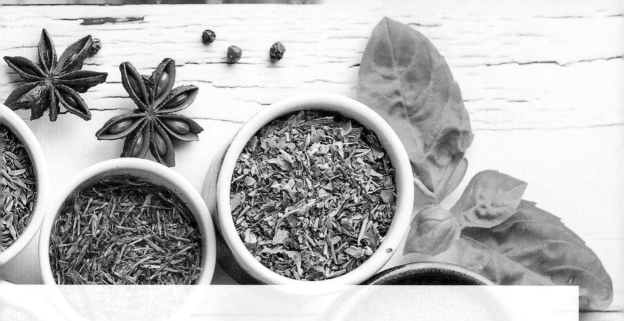

culinary masterpiece that is both delicious and enhances your health.

Culinary herbs and spices contain high concentrations of unique phytochemicals that can alter metabolic and cellular processes with potentially positive clinical effects. The richest sources of polyphenols are spices and herbs: herbs of the Lamiaceae family – peppermint, sage, rosemary, spearmint, thyme – contain the highest amounts of a powerful antioxidant compound, hydroxycinnamic acid.

Cloves, peppermint and star anise comprise the highest concentrations of phenolic compounds (eugenol in cloves, eriocitrin in peppermint and anethole in star anise), followed by oregano, sage and rosemary.

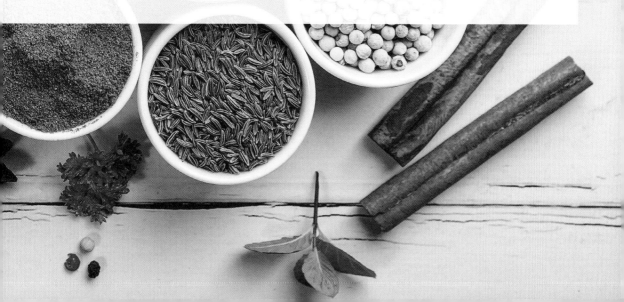

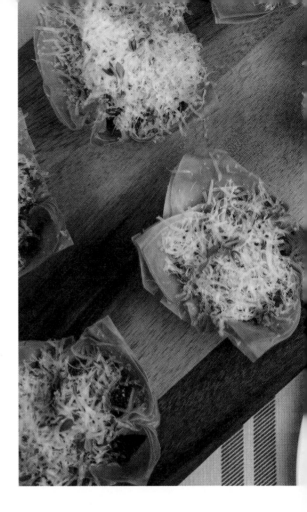

Ratatouille filo cups with parmesan

SERVES 4

350 g filo pastry (defrost if frozen)

3 tablespoons extra virgin olive oil

1 small eggplant, cut into 1 cm (½ in) dice

2 zucchini (courgette), cut into 1 cm (½ in) dice

1 medium onion, cut into 1 cm (½ in) dice

2 small yellow capsicums, cut into 1 cm (½ in) dice

3 garlic cloves, finely chopped

1½ tablespoons tomato paste

1 tablespoon thyme leaves, chopped

½ tablespoon smoked paprika

¼ teaspoon cayenne

3 medium tomatoes, cut into 1 cm (½ in) dice

80 g (2¾ oz) grated parmesan

salt and pepper to taste

Preheat the oven to 160°C (320°F).

You will need a 12-cup non-stick muffin tray. Create a guide for the filo squares by cutting a baking paper square to size, large enough to fill the mould.

Unfold the filo pastry and cover with a slightly damp cloth. Take one sheet at a time and lightly brush with extra virgin olive oil. Repeat with two more sheets, then stack the three oiled sheets together. Repeat the process to create four stacks of sheets, being careful to keep the stacks separate and cover them to prevent them from drying out. Using the paper guide, cut 12 squares from the stacks of sheets. Line each mould with a single stack of pastry.

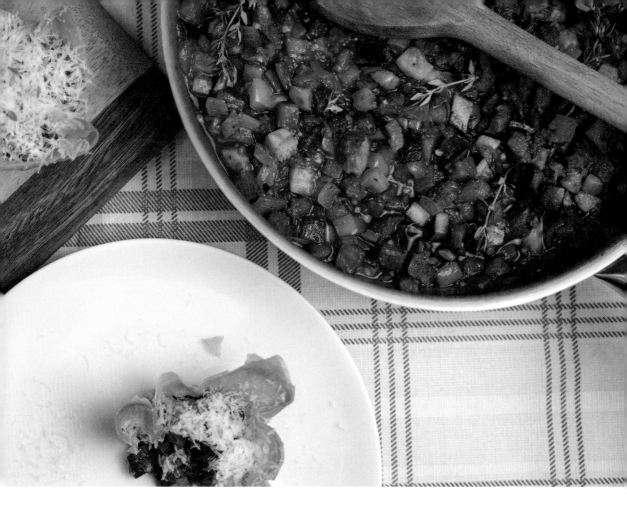

Bake for 12–15 minutes. Carefully remove the filo cups and place on a rack to cool.

Heat 1 tablespoon of extra virgin olive oil in a large non-stick frying pan over a medium heat. Add the eggplant and season with salt. Cook, stirring frequently, until soft and starting to brown, for 10 minutes approximately. Set aside in a bowl. Add another tablespoon of oil to the pan and add the zucchini and cook until tender, 3–4 minutes. Season and transfer to a bowl.

Add the last tablespoons of oil to the pan and add the onion and capsicum. Cook, stirring frequently, for about 5 minutes until the onion has softened. Add the garlic and continue cooking for about 1 more minute without browning. Add the tomato paste, thyme, paprika and cayenne. Cook for a further 1–2 minutes while stirring. Now add the diced tomatoes and continue to cook over a medium heat, stirring occasionally, until the tomatoes have broken down, about 8–10 minutes. Return the cooked eggplant to the pan, bring to heat and simmer, uncovered, for about 10 minutes. Add the sautéed zucchini and cook for 1–2 minutes more, or until fully heated through. Taste and adjust seasoning if necessary.

Spoon the mixture in the filo cups and top with grated parmesan to serve.

Mushroom carnitas tacos

SERVES 4

FOR THE PICO DE GALLO
1 small red onion

2 large tomatoes

1 small capsicum

1 deseeded jalapeno, finely chopped

½ bunch coriander, (cilantro) chopped

1 lime, juiced

½ tablespoon extra virgin olive oil

salt and pepper to taste

FOR THE TORTILLAS
330 g (1 oz) wholemeal baker's flour

1 teaspoon salt

1 teaspoon baking powder

180 ml (6 fl oz) warm water

1 teaspoon honey

60 ml (2 fl oz) extra virgin olive oil

FOR THE CARNITAS
600 g (1 lb 5 oz) king brown mushrooms

1 large brown onion, finely sliced

1½ tablespoons extra virgin olive oil

4 garlic cloves, finely chopped

1 teaspoon ground coriander

1½ teaspoons ground cumin

1½ teaspoons smoked paprika

1 teaspoon dried oregano

1 bay leaf

2 tablespoons chipotle peppers in adobo sauce, chopped

1 tablespoon tomato paste

350 ml (12 fl oz) water

1 orange, juiced

zest of ½ orange

salt and pepper to taste

Guacamole (page 184)

3 tablespoons low-fat natural yoghurt

½ bunch fresh coriander (cilantro), picked leaves

For the pico de gallo, finely dice the onion, tomato and capsicum. Fold through the remaining ingredients, transfer into a serving bowl, cover and place in the fridge.

For the tortillas, place the flour, salt and baking powder in a bowl and mix. Form a well in the centre and set aside. In a separate bowl mix together the water, honey and oil. Pour the liquid into the centre of the dry ingredients and stir from the centre to mix the dry and wet ingredients to form a dough. Once a dough is formed, knead vigorously for 5 minutes until it is smooth, silky and elastic.

Divide into 8 to 10 equal pieces and shape into balls with the palm of your hand. Cover the balls with a slightly damp cloth and rest for 20–30 minutes.

In the meantime, cut the stem off the mushrooms and finely slice the caps. Using your fingers pull apart the stems of the mushrooms to resemble strands of pulled pork.

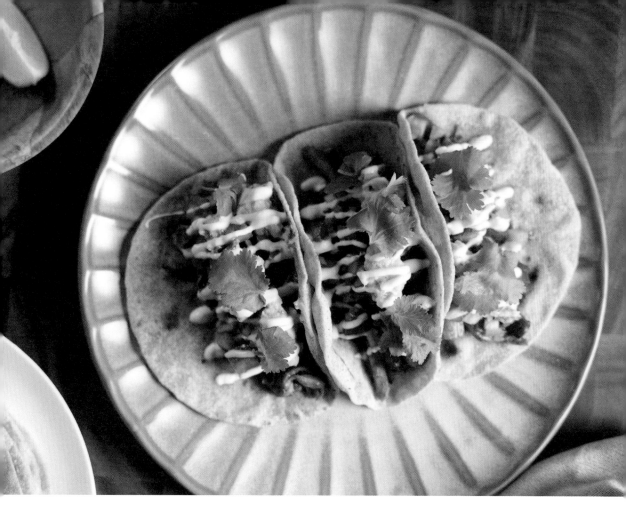

Set a heavy pan on medium–high heat. Working in batches sauté the mushrooms and onion in olive oil until the onion is soft and mushrooms are slightly browned. Once they are done, lower the heat and return all the mushrooms and onions to the pan. Add the garlic and cook for a further 1 or 2 minutes while stirring – don't brown the garlic.

Next add the spices, oregano and bay leaf, cook for a further 1 minute while stirring.

Add the chipotle and tomato paste, and cook for a further minute.

Lastly add the water, orange juice and zest. Season to taste. Bring the pan to a simmer, cover and cook for 20–30 minutes.

Once the dough has rested, lightly flour a bench and, using a rolling pin, roll each ball into a flat disc 2–3 mm (⅛ in) thick, making sure the dough doesn't stick.

Heat a large frying pan over a high heat and cook each tortilla (no oil added) until it bubbles and the bottom is slightly coloured. Flip over and cook for a further 30–40 seconds. Set aside on a plate ready to serve.

To serve, set out bowls of guacamole, pico de gallo and carnitas with a plate of tortillas and allow each person to construct their own tacos at the table. Garnish with a dollop of yoghurt and coriander leaves.

Buckwheat sourdough blinis with lentil caponata and labneh

SERVES 4

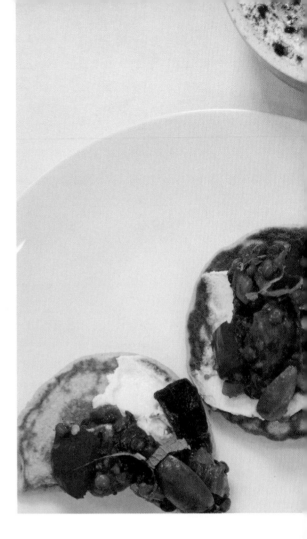

FOR THE BLINIS

200 ml (7 fl oz) milk

80 g (2¾ oz) sourdough starter

½ teaspoon baker's yeast

¼ teaspoon honey

110 g (4 oz) wholemeal flour

60 g (2 oz) buckwheat flour

½ teaspoon salt

FOR THE CAPONATA

600 g (1lb 5 oz) eggplant, cut into
   1½ cm (½ in) dice

4 tablespoons extra virgin olive oil

400 g (14 oz) red capsicum, diced

150 g (5½ oz) brown onion, diced

150 g (5½ oz) celery, diced

2 cloves garlic, minced

400 g (14 oz) canned chopped tomatoes

80 g (2¾ oz) green olives, pitted and sliced

80 g (2¾ oz) kalamata olives, pitted and sliced

40 g (1½ oz) capers, drained

55 ml (1¾ fl oz) white wine vinegar

20 g (¾ oz) honey

200 g (7 oz) cooked green lentils

2½ cups/45 g (1½ oz) basil leaves, sliced

salt and pepper to taste

Labneh (page 184)

Preheat the oven to 220°C (430°F). To make the blini batter, warm the milk and place in a mixing bowl. Add the sourdough starter, yeast and honey. Whisk until well combined. Sieve the flours into the milk mixture and add the salt. Using a wooden spoon or a spatula mix the flour and milk mixture until well combined and lump free. Do not overmix. Cover and place in the fridge.

For the caponata, mix the eggplant in a bowl with 2 tablespoons of olive oil and salt and pepper to taste. Transfer to a lined baking tray and bake for 10 minutes. Turn the cubes and cook for a further 10 minutes. Reduce the oven temperature to 180°C (350°F). Add the

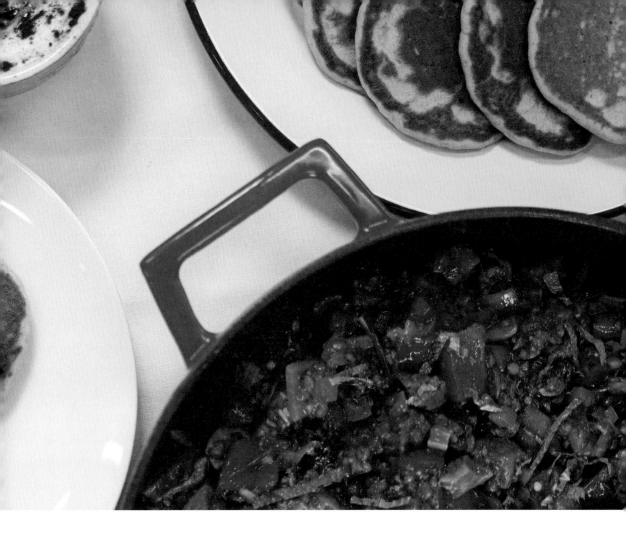

capsicum to the tray with 1 tablespoon of olive oil and cook for another 20 minutes, turning the vegetables after 10.

In the meantime, place the remaining tablespoon of olive oil in a large frying pan and warm over a medium heat. Sweat the onion and celery, stirring occasionally, until cooked through and translucent. Add the garlic and cook for a further minute. Add the tomatoes, olives, capers, vinegar and honey. Cover and cook over a low heat for 10 minutes. Remove the lid and add the capsicum and eggplant. Season to taste and cook for a further 5 minutes. Fold through the lentils and basil. Set aside.

To cook the blinis, place a large non-stick frying pan over a medium heat. Lightly coat the surface of the pan with olive oil using a piece of kitchen paper. Once the pan is hot, add spoonfuls of batter (about 1 tablespoon for a 6–7 cm blini) to the pan, cooking two or three at a time. Cook until bubbles start to form on the surface and the underside of the blinis has browned. Carefully flip them and cook for a further minute. Repeat this process until all the batter has been used. Serve the hot blinis topped with caponata and a dollop of labneh.

Burghul savoury cake with epityrum and roasted tomatoes

SERVES 4

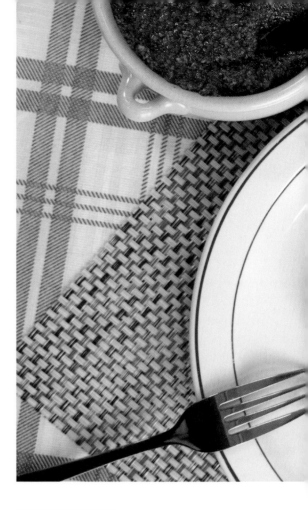

200 g (7 oz) cherry tomatoes

1 tablespoon extra virgin olive oil

salt and pepper

FOR THE CAKE

400 g (14 oz) fine burghul wheat

60 g (2 oz) frozen peas

60 g (2 oz) frozen corn kernels

120 g (4½ oz) carrot, finely grated

120 g (4½ oz) red onion, finely chopped

400 g (14 oz) ricotta

30 ml (1 fl oz) extra virgin olive oil

1 teaspoon smoked paprika

8 g (¼ oz) salt

1 teaspoon baking soda

1 teaspoon baking powder

200 ml (7 fl oz) water

2 tablespoons white sesame seeds

2 tablespoons black sesame seeds

FOR THE EPITYRUM

120 g (4½ oz) green olives, pitted

120 g (4½ oz) kalamata olives, pitted

1 teaspoon ground cumin

½ teaspoon ground fennel seed

1 cup rocket arugula) leaves, loosely packed

½ cup mint leaves, loosely packed

80 ml (2½ fl oz) extra virgin olive oil

20 ml (¾ fl oz) white wine vinegar

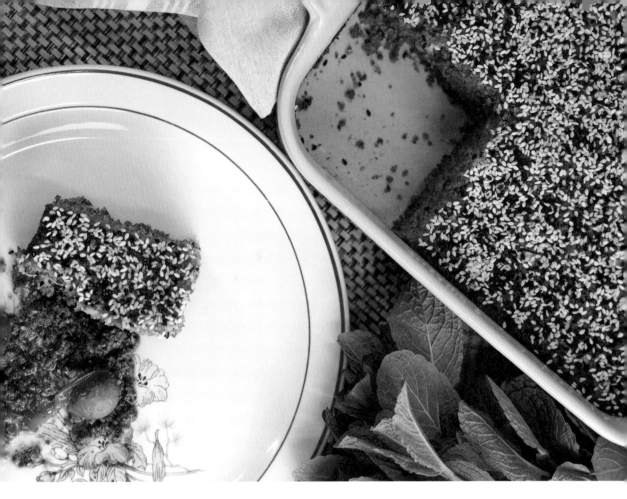

Preheat the oven to 180°C (350°F). In a medium bowl, dress the cherry tomatoes with salt, pepper and a drizzle of olive oil. Place on a baking tray and bake until the skin is slightly shrivelled but not collapsing, about 8–10 minutes. Remove from the tray and set aside.

Place all the cake ingredients, except the sesame seeds, in a large bowl. Mix until the mixture is well combined. Spoon into a 25 cm (10 in) cake tin. Top with sesame seeds and bake for 35–40 minutes or until a skewer inserted comes out clean. Remove from oven to cool slightly.

In the meantime, for the epityrum, place all the ingredients in a food processor. Process until smooth.

Serve the cake in slices with a dollop of epityrum and the roasted tomatoes.

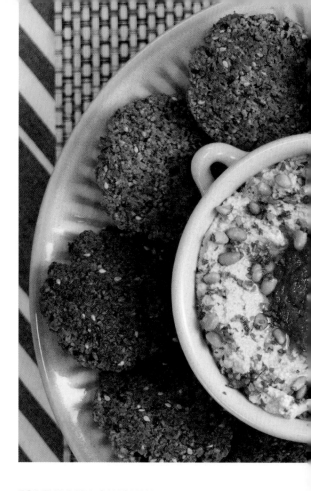

Baked falafel with baba ganoush and harissa

SERVES 4

FOR THE FALAFEL
150 g (5½ oz) dried chickpeas

30 g (1 oz) two-day-old bread (no crusts)

½ cup milk

30 g (1 oz) finely chopped parsley

1 medium onion, finely diced

3 garlic cloves, finely chopped

½ teaspoon ground cumin

½ teaspoon ground coriander

½ teaspoon baking powder

1 teaspoon nutritional yeast

1½ tablespoons sesame seeds

½ teaspoon salt

20 ml (¾ fl oz) extra virgin olive oil

FOR THE BABA GANOUSH
3 large eggplants (about 1 kg/2 lb total)

125 g (4½ oz) tahini

2 garlic cloves

1 lemon juiced

40 g (1½ oz) natural yoghurt

45 ml (1½ fl oz) extra virgin olive oil

½ teaspoon ground cumin

½ teaspoon ground coriander

½ teaspoon paprika

salt and pepper to taste

30 g (1 oz) harissa

1 tablespoon pine nuts, toasted

1 tablespoon coriander (cilantro) leaves, chopped

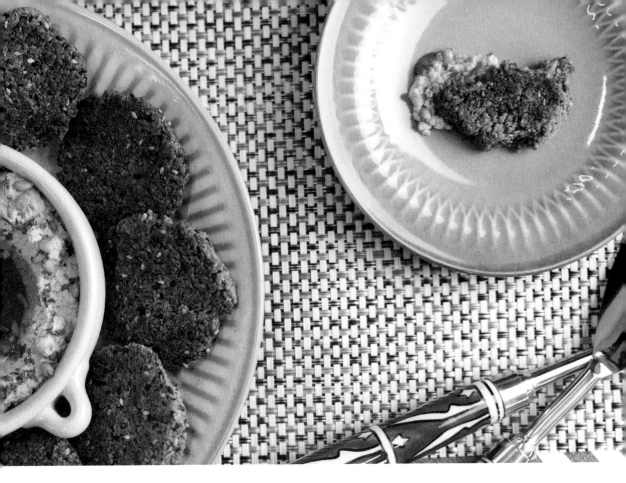

The day before planning to serve the falafel, soak the chickpeas in plenty of water and place in the fridge. The next day, drain the chickpeas well, place in a food processor and process until it reaches a couscous-like texture. Transfer to a large bowl and set aside.

Using a skewer, prick small holes in the eggplants and place over a live gas or barbecue flame. Char well on all sides until the skin is blistered (about 5–7 minutes each side) and the inside is cooked. Place in a bowl and cover with cling wrap. Leave to cool, then scoop out the flesh and discard the skin.

For the falafel, preheat the oven to 180°C (350°F). Soak the stale bread in the milk until it is well softened. Squeeze out the milk and place the bread in the bowl with the chickpea mix. Add the remaining falafel ingredients and mix well, using your hands. Make sure the bread is well broken down and all the ingredients are evenly combined. Divide the mix into 12 disks and place onto a lined and slightly oiled baking sheet. Bake for 25–30 minutes, turning the falafel over halfway through.

In the meantime, process the eggplant with all the remaining baba ganoush ingredients in a blender until smooth. Transfer to a serving bowl and top with harissa, pine nuts and coriander. Serve the falafel with a generous portion of baba ganoush.

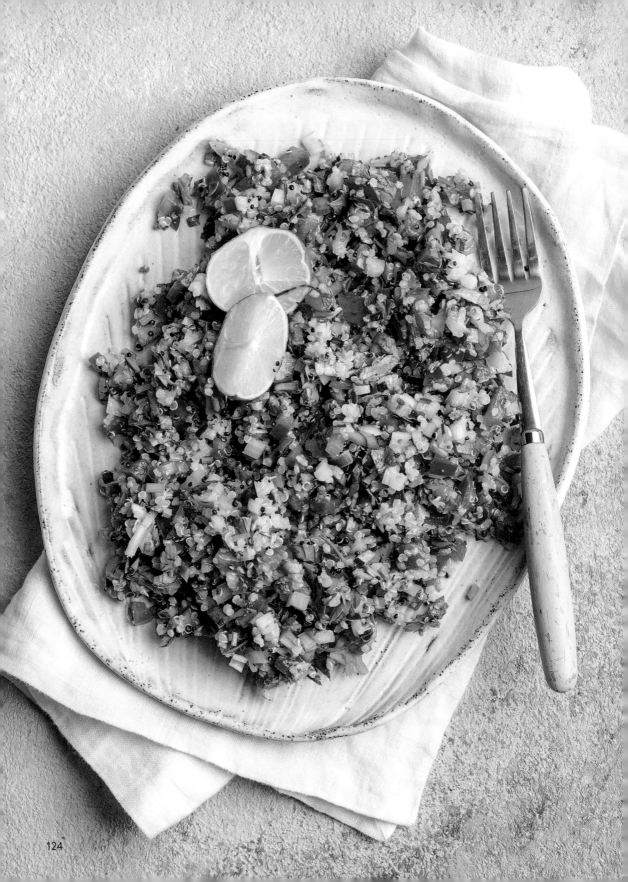

Mains

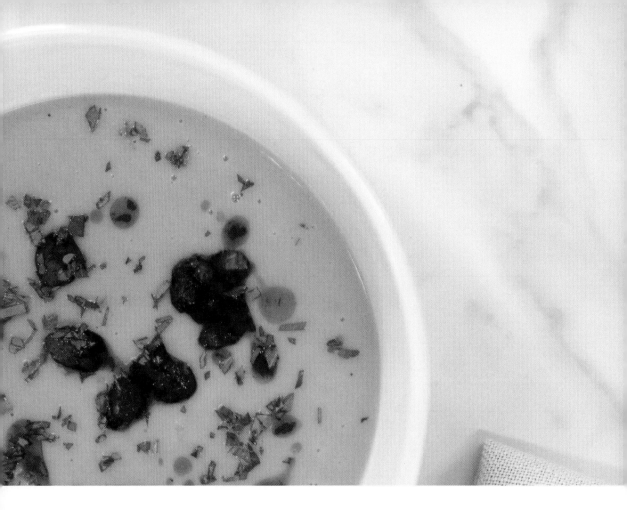

White bean and cauliflower soup with chilli oil

SERVES 4

1 tablespoon extra virgin olive oil

1 small onion, roughly diced

1 medium carrot, roughly diced

1 large celery stick, roughly diced

4 cloves garlic, crushed

50 g (1¾ oz) white miso paste

180 ml (6 fl oz) white wine

400 g (14 oz) cauliflower florets

350 g (12½ oz) cooked white navy beans

1 litre (34 fl oz) vegetable stock

3–4 thyme sprigs

1–2 bay leaves

salt and pepper to taste

FOR THE CHILLI OIL

40 ml (1¼ fl oz) extra virgin olive oil

30 g (1 oz) fermented chilli paste or sambal oelek

30 g (1 oz) toasted almonds, crushed or finely chopped

1 tablespoon lemon juice

2 tablespoons chopped parsley

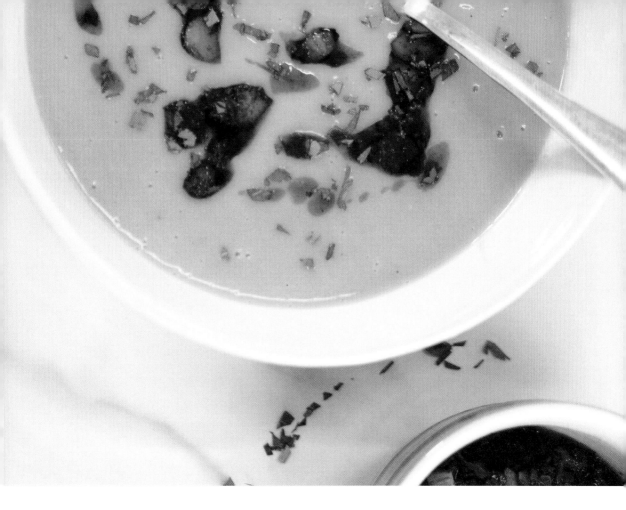

Heat 1 tablespoon of olive oil in a large saucepan over a medium heat. Add the onion, carrot, and celery. Cook gently without the vegetables gaining colour and until the onion is translucent, about 5 minutes. Add the garlic and cook for a further 2 minutes while stirring.

Add the miso and wine and stir well. Cook until the liquid reduces and the wine has evaporated.

Add the cauliflower, beans, stock, thyme and bay leaf to the pan. Season with salt and pepper. Bring to a simmer, partly covering with a lid, and cook until the cauliflower is tender.

In the meantime, in a small saucepan combine the olive oil, chilli paste and nuts. Bring to a simmer over a low heat. Cook for 2 minutes until fragrant, then remove from the heat and add the lemon juice.

Discard the bay leaves from the soup and blend with a hand-held blender until smooth. Season to taste. Bring back to heat, then transfer to serving bowls, garnish with the chilli oil and parsley and serve immediately.

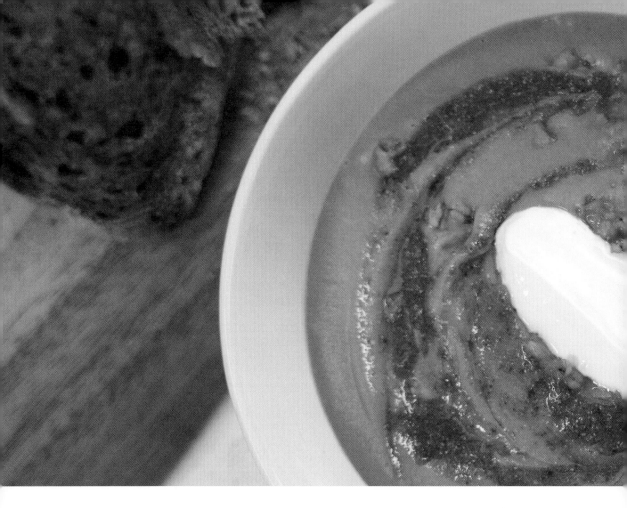

Split pea and spinach soup with barley and mint pesto

SERVES 4

1 tablespoon extra virgin olive oil

2 large leeks, finely sliced

1 celery stick, finely sliced

3 garlic cloves

2 litres (68 fl oz) vegetable stock

200 g (7 oz) dried split peas

1 bay leaf

salt and pepper to taste

150 g (1¾ oz) spinach, washed

100 g (3½ oz) cooked pearl barley

4 tablespoons low-fat natural yoghurt

FOR THE PESTO

1 garlic clove

¼ cup pine nuts, toasted

¼ cup extra virgin olive oil

1½ cups mint leaves, loosely packed

1 cup parsley leaves, loosely packed

⅛ teaspoon chilli flakes

1–2 tablespoons fresh lemon juice to taste

salt and pepper to taste

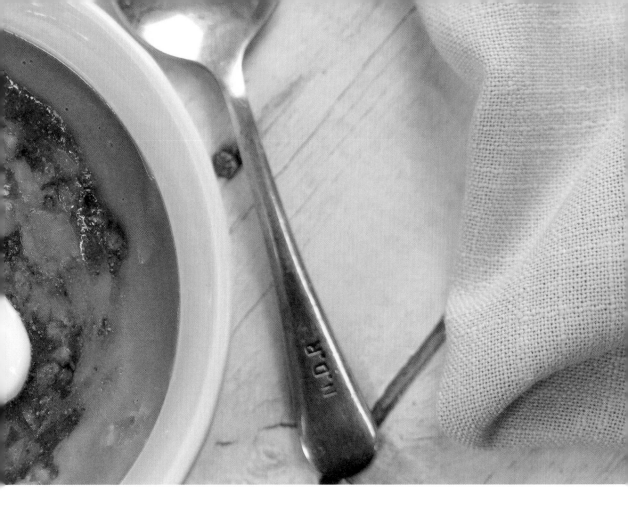

In a large saucepan, heat the olive oil over a medium heat and add the leek, celery and garlic. Stir frequently in order to prevent any colour forming; turn down the heat if cooking too quickly. Once softened, add the stock and split peas. Bring to a simmer and add the bay leaf, then salt and pepper to taste. Cook for about 20 minutes until the split peas are tender but not mushy. Once the peas are cooked, remove the bay leaf and take the saucepan off the heat. Stir through the spinach until it wilts.

Process the soup with a hand-held blender in the saucepan or in a blender in batches. Adjust for seasoning and reheat if necessary.

To prepare the mint pesto, blend the garlic, pine nuts and olive oil using a food processor or blender. When well blended add the mint and parsley and process until smooth. Fold through the chilli flakes and add lemon juice to taste. Season with salt and pepper.

Serve the soup topped with pearl barley, mint pesto and a dollop of yoghurt.

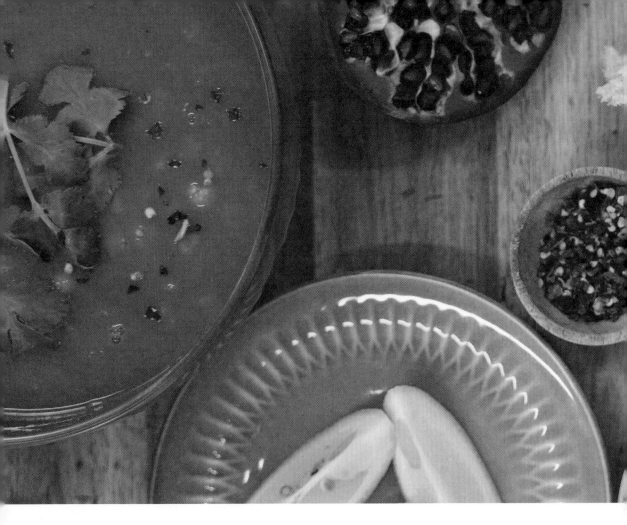

Tunisian chickpea soup (Lablabi)

SERVES 4

2 tablespoons extra virgin olive oil

1 small carrot, finely diced

1 celery stick, finely diced

1 small onion, finely diced

3 garlic cloves, finely chopped

1½ teaspoons ground cumin

1½ teaspoons ground coriander

1½ teaspoons smoked paprika

1 tablespoon harissa

1 tablespoon tomato paste

480 g (2¾ oz) cooked chickpeas

1 litre (34 fl oz) vegetable stock

50 g (1¾ oz) low-fat Greek yoghurt

1 handful coriander (cilantro) leaves, picked

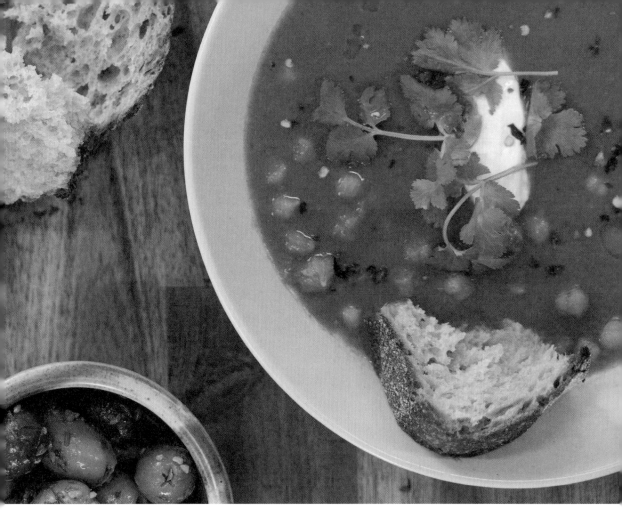

Heat the olive oil in a large saucepan over a medium heat. Add the carrot, celery and onion. Cook gently without the vegetables gaining colour and until the onion is translucent. Add the garlic and cook for a further 2 minutes, stirring all the time.

Add the spices and stir well for about 1 minute, being careful not to burn them. Add the harissa and tomato paste and cook for a further minute.

Finally add the chickpeas and stock. Reduce to a low simmer, partly covering the pan with a lid, and cook until all the vegetables are tender and the soup has thickened (about 20–30 minutes). Set aside to cool a little, then use a hand-held blender to liquidise well. Return soup to heat and season to taste. Serve with a dollop of yoghurt and garnish with coriander.

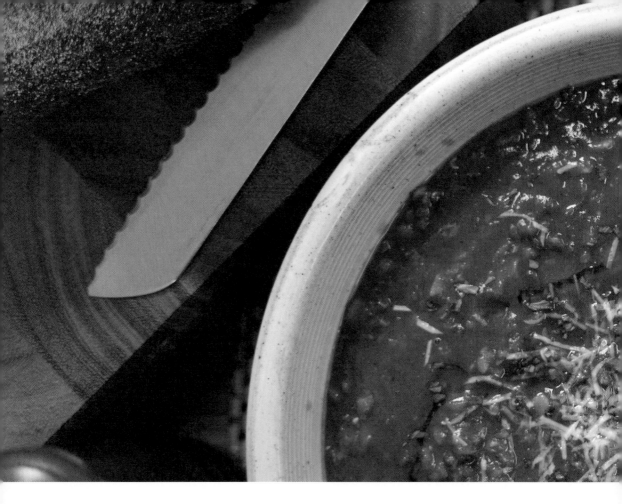

Mixed lentil soup

SERVES 4

2 tablespoons extra virgin olive oil

1 medium carrot, finely diced

1 small onion, finely diced

2 celery sticks, finely diced

2 garlic cloves, finely chopped

2 teaspoons dried marjoram

1 teaspoon ground allspice

1 tablespoon tomato paste

1 litre (34 fl oz) vegetable stock

400 g (14 oz) can crushed tomatoes

250 g (9 oz) mixed lentils

1 bay leaf

1 parmesan rind (optional)

2 tablespoons grated parmesan

2 tablespoons flat-leaf parsley, chopped

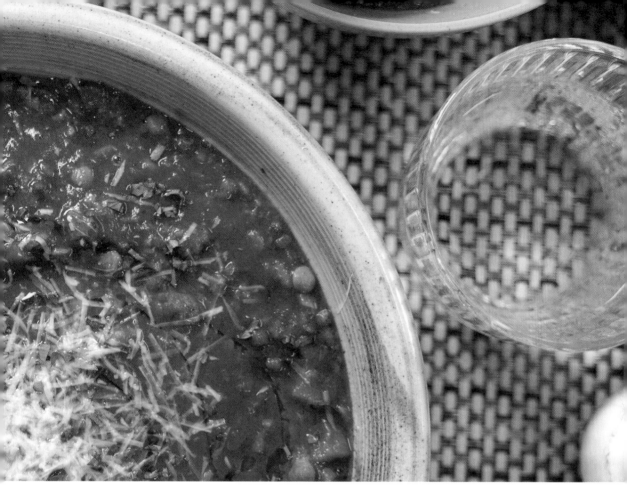

Heat the oil in a large pot over a medium heat. Add the carrot, onion and celery. Sweat for a few minutes until the onion is translucent. Add the garlic, marjoram and allspice. Cook for a further 2 minutes while stirring. Add tomato paste and cook for another 2 minutes, stirring all the time. Now add the stock, crushed tomatoes, lentils, bay leaf and parmesan rind (if using). Season to taste and bring to a simmer. Slowly simmer until all the lentils are cooked through, about 20 minutes. If the soup is too thick add a little water.

Serve hot in individual bowls, garnished with parsley and parmesan.

Winter farro power bowl with avocado cream and sprouts

SERVES 4

2 bunches Dutch carrots (about 12)

500 g (1 lb 2 oz) sweet potato, cut into
    2 cm (½ in) dice

1 tablespoon extra virgin olive oil

200 g (7 oz) kale, thinly sliced

2 cups alfalfa sprouts

2 cups snow pea sprouts

150 g (5½ oz) cooked farro

240 g (8½ oz) cooked chickpeas

salt and pepper to taste

FOR THE PICKLED CABBAGE

350 g (12½ oz) red cabbage, thinly sliced

35 ml (1¼ fl oz) apple cider vinegar

2 teaspoons honey

¼ teaspoon celery seeds

⅛ teaspoon sumac

¼ teaspoon salt

FOR THE AVOCADO CREAM

2 medium avocados

35 ml (1¼ fl oz) lime juice

1 tablespoon extra virgin olive oil

salt and pepper to taste

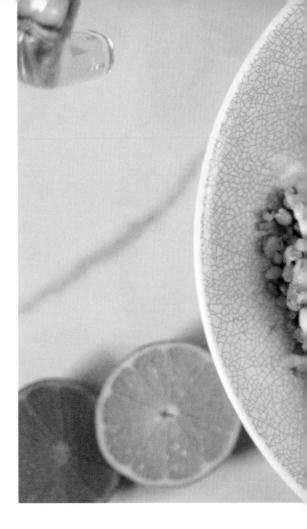

FOR THE TAHINI DRESSING

80 g (2¾ oz) tahini

45 ml (1½ fl oz) lemon juice

2 teaspoons honey

¼ teaspoon salt

½ garlic clove, minced

90 ml (3 fl oz) water

Preheat the oven to 200°C (400°F). Wash
the carrots well and trim the stems. Toss the
carrots and sweet potato in a mixing bowl with
2 tablespoons of olive oil, then season with salt
and pepper to taste. Transfer to a baking sheet
and place in the oven. Roast for 20–25 minutes
or until done. Set aside.

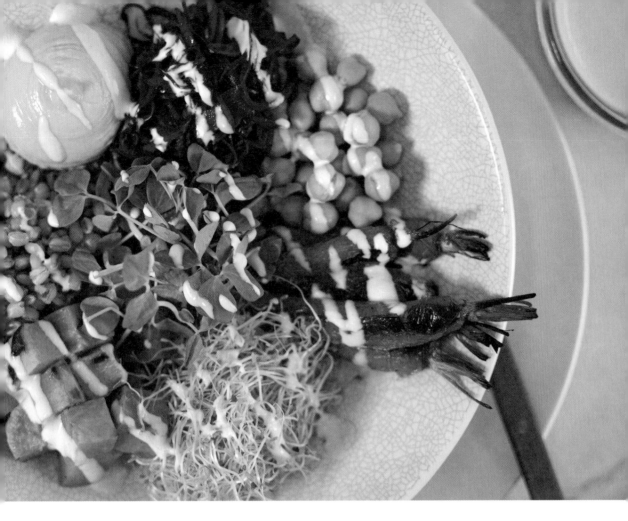

In the meantime, mix the cabbage with the vinegar, honey, celery seeds, sumac and salt in a large bowl and refrigerate for 2 hours, mixing it every 30 minutes.

For the avocado cream, place the avocado, lime juice and olive oil in a blender and season with salt and pepper. Blitz until smooth then transfer to a small bowl.

Combine and whisk all the ingredients for the tahini dressing together until well combined.

Place the kale in a mixing bowl with 2 tablespoons of the tahini dressing. Use your hands to soften the kale a little, squeezing it between your fingers as you mix in the dressing.

To assemble, place a portion of kale in the bottom of four serving bowls. Sit the sprouts in the centre and arrange the sweet potato, carrots, farro, chickpeas and red cabbage around them, keeping each element separate. Dot the bowl with avocado cream, drizzle with more tahini dressing and serve.

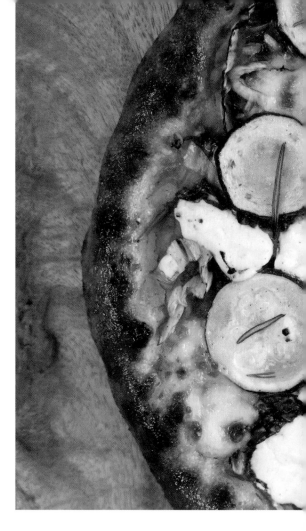

Wholemeal pizza with pumpkin, radicchio, zucchini, walnuts and goat's cheese

SERVES 4

FOR THE DOUGH
600 g (1 lb 5 oz) strong wholemeal flour

13 g (½ oz) salt

440 ml (15 fl oz) water

30 ml (1 fl oz) extra virgin olive oil

½ teaspoon baker's yeast

130 g (4½ oz) sourdough starter or additional
  ¼ teaspoon baker's yeast

1 teaspoon honey

400 g (14 oz) pumpkin, diced

1 small radicchio, shredded

3 medium zucchini (courgette), sliced in thin rounds

50 g (1¾ oz) toasted walnuts, crushed

200 g (7 oz) goat's cheese

1 sprig of rosemary

2 tablespoons extra virgin olive oil

To make the dough, ideally start the day before. Place the flour and salt in a large bowl. Mix well and form a well in the middle. Place the water, oil, yeast, sourdough starter and honey in a separate bowl. Mix thoroughly and allow to stand for 2 minutes.

Pour the sourdough and yeast mixture into the flour. Slowly start to mix the ingredients, from the outer rim towards the centre, using a wooden spoon or your hands. Keep mixing until a dough has formed. Transfer onto a lightly floured bench and knead for 2–3 minutes until it is stretchy and well combined. Wipe the bowl of any residue and brush the inside lightly with olive oil. Place the dough back in the bowl,

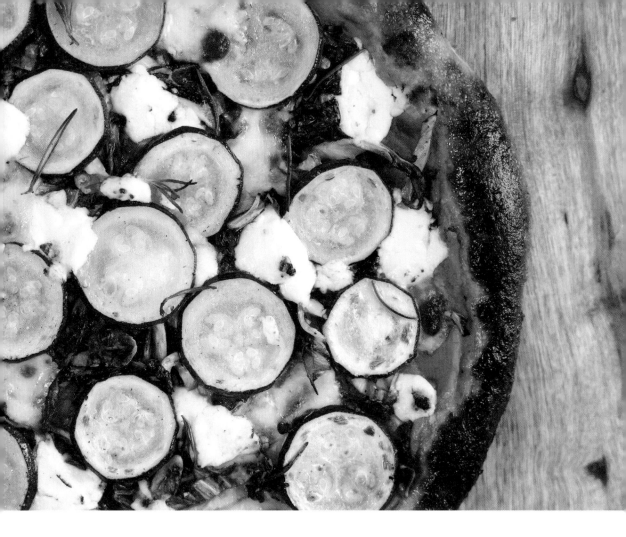

cover with cling wrap and refrigerate overnight (or from 6–24 hours).

The next day, preheat the oven to 200°C (400°F). Portion the dough into four 250 g (9 oz) pieces, rolling and shaping them gently into balls with your hands. Place the balls on a lightly floured tray and cover with a damp cloth. Place in a warm area until the dough has doubled in size.

Toss the pumpkin in a mixing bowl with 1 tablespoon of olive oil, then season with salt and pepper to taste. Transfer to a baking sheet and place in the oven. Roast for 15–20 minutes or until done. Set aside.

Roll out the pizza dough into circles and top with the roasted pumpkin, radicchio, zucchini, walnuts, goat's cheese and sprigs of roasemary. Drizzle with olive oil and bake for 20–30 minutes or until the the pizza is golden brown.

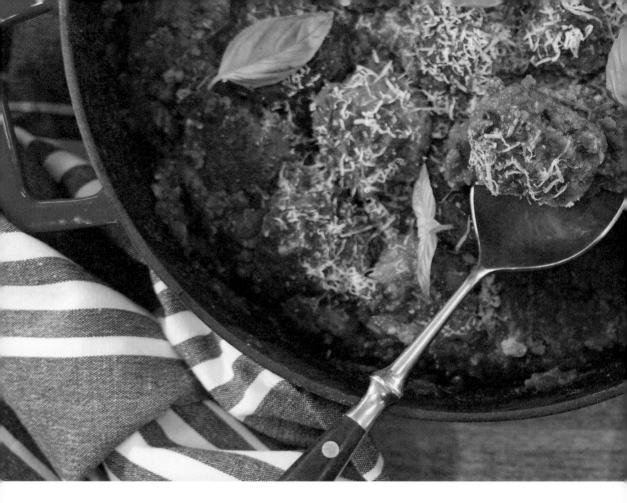

Vegetarian meatballs

SERVES 4

115 g (4 oz) brown rice
500 g (1 lb 2 oz) brown mushrooms
3 tablespoons extra virgin olive oil
1 medium onion, finely diced
3 garlic cloves, minced
1 tablespoon thyme leaves
250 g (9 oz) grated cauliflower
2 tablespoons tomato paste
1 tablespoon nutritional yeast
1 teaspoon porcini powder (optional)
35 g (1¼ oz) grated parmesan

35 g (1¼ oz) breadcrumbs
2 teaspoons seeded mustard
2 eggs
ground nutmeg to taste
salt and pepper to taste
wholemeal flour as needed
1 litre (34 fl oz) tomato sugo (page 140)

Place the rice in a medium saucepan of boiling salted water and simmer, stirring regularly, until the rice is slightly overcooked, about 60–70 minutes. Drain well and set aside.

In the meantime, finely chop the mushrooms and heat a large frying pan over high heat. Add 1 tablespoon of olive oil to the pan and

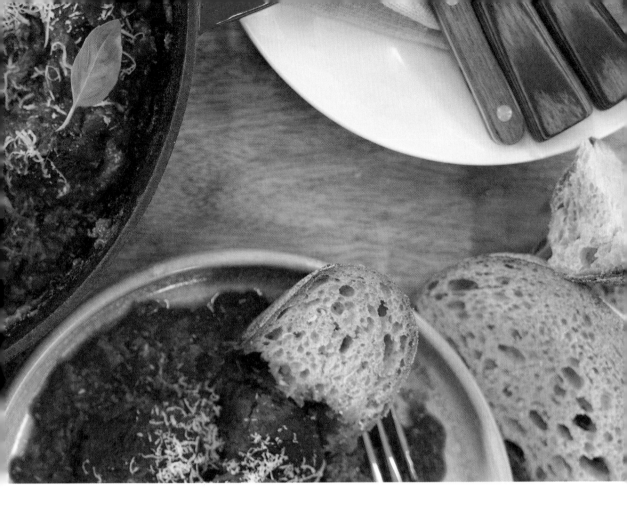

add the mushrooms. Cook until well coloured and quite dry, reducing the heat if required so as not to burn the mushrooms. Remove the mushrooms and set aside.

Heat 1 tablespoon of olive oil in the frying pan and sauté the onion over a low heat, stirring gently, until well coloured and soft. Add the garlic and thyme and cook for a further 2 minutes.

Put the mushrooms, rice and onion mix in a food processor (working in batches) and pulse until the consistency of minced meat. Transfer the mix to a bowl and add all the remaining ingredients, except for the flour and sugo. Combine well.

Using slightly wet hands form the mixture into meatball-sized balls and transfer to a tray. Place uncovered in the fridge for 2 hours to chill. Once cold, roll each ball in wholemeal flour, shaking off any excess. Place a large frying pan over a medium heat, and using the last tablespoon of olive oil cook the meatballs until well coloured on all sides. Turn the balls gently to retain their shape.

Once all the meatballs are sealed and coloured, remove from the pan. Wipe the pan clean, pour in the tomato sugo and gently add the meatballs. Cook over a low heat until the sauce has reduced a little and the meatballs are hot.

Spinach and ricotta tortelloni with tomato sugo

SERVES 4

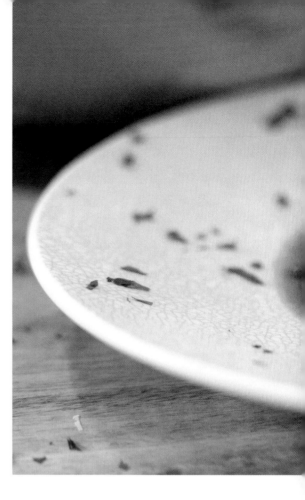

FOR THE TOMATO SUGO
2 tablespoons extra virgin olive oil

4 garlic cloves, halved

1 small brown onion, finely chopped

1 tablespoon tomato paste

2 × 400 g (14 oz) cans chopped tomatoes

1 handful basil leaves, torn (plus extra for garnish)

salt and pepper to taste

FOR THE PASTA
300 g (10½ oz) wholemeal flour

100 g (3½ oz) fine semolina

4 eggs

1 tablespoon extra virgin olive oil

80 ml (2½ fl oz) water

pinch of salt

FOR THE FILLING
600 g (1 lb 5 oz) ricotta, drained of all whey

300 g (10½ oz) cooked (or frozen) spinach,
    finely chopped and well squeezed

2 eggs

130 g (4½ oz) grated parmesan (plus extra
    to serve)

ground nutmeg to taste

salt and pepper to taste

In a medium-sized, heavy-bottomed saucepan heat 2 tablespoons of olive oil over a low heat. Add the garlic and cook until slightly coloured. Remove and discard. Add the onion and cook until translucent. Add the tomato paste and cook for a further minute. Lastly add the tomatoes and basil. Season with salt and pepper. Bring the sugo to a slow simmer and cook, half covered, for 2–4 hours or until it is thick and rich. Stir frequently to avoid it sticking.

To make the pasta dough, combine the flour, semolina, 4 eggs, 1 tablespoon extra virgin olive oil, water and salt in a bowl. Mix until a firm dough is formed. Transfer to a bench and knead until the dough becomes silky and well mixed. Cover with cling wrap and place in the fridge to rest for 2–12 hours.

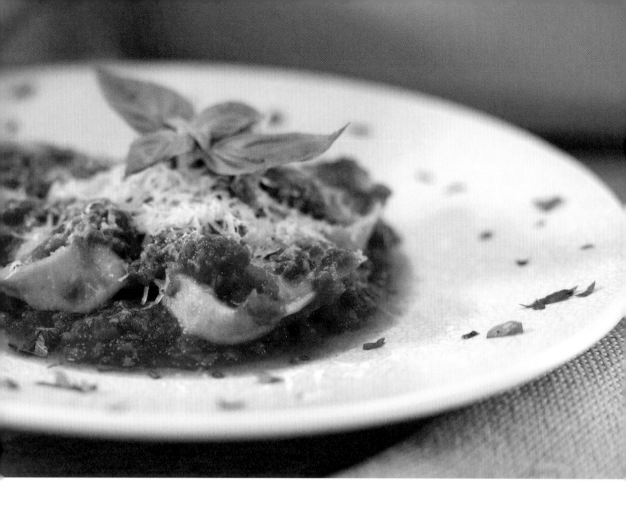

In the meantime, prepare the filling. In a medium bowl, mix together the well-drained ricotta, spinach, 2 eggs and parmesan. Season with nutmeg, salt and pepper.

Using a pasta machine or a rolling pin, roll the pasta dough until your hand can be seen from the other side when placed against the pasta dough, about 1½ mm (⅛ in) thickness.

Working in batches, cut the sheet in 7 cm (2¾ in) squares while keeping the rest of the dough covered with a slightly damp cloth.

Place 1 heaped teaspoon of the ricotta mixture in the middle of each square. Lightly wet two of the four sides using a brush. Fold the square into a triangle, over the ricotta mix,

pressing the edges together at the same time as squeezing out any air.

Take the bottom corners of the triangle, pinching the ends together to form a tortellini shape. Repeat this until the filling or pasta dough has been used up.

Put a large pot of salted water on a high heat and bring to the boil. Drop in batches of the tortelloni, stirring gently so they don't stick together. Cook until they float and the thickest area of pasta is cooked (about 2–3 minutes).

While the tortelloni are cooking, return the sugo to heat. Divide the tortelloni among 4 serving bowls, topped with the tomato sugo. Serve immediately with parmesan and some basil leaves.

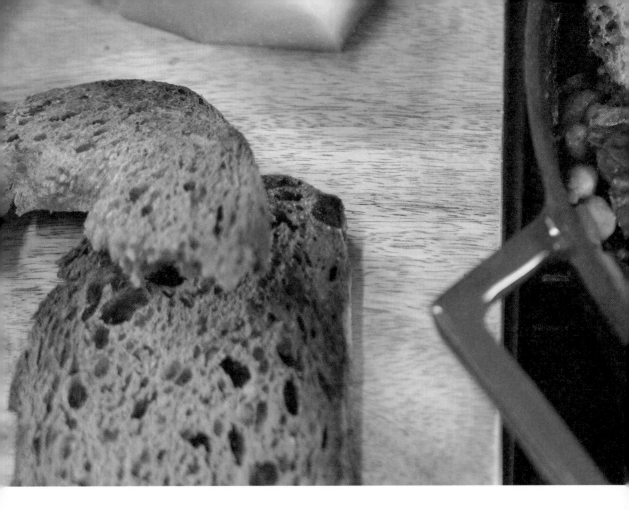

Spicy chickpeas with tomatoes and winter greens

SERVES 4

2 tablespoons extra virgin olive oil

1 small brown onion, diced

2 garlic cloves, crushed

1 teaspoon fresh ginger, minced

1½ teaspoons Madras curry powder

1 tablespoon tomato paste

1 tablespoon red miso paste

400 g (14 oz) can chopped tomatoes

480 g (2¾ oz) cooked chickpeas

150 ml (5 fl oz) vegetable stock

150 g (1¾ oz) silverbeet leaves (stems removed), coarsely chopped

grated parmesan (optional)

wholemeal bread, to serve

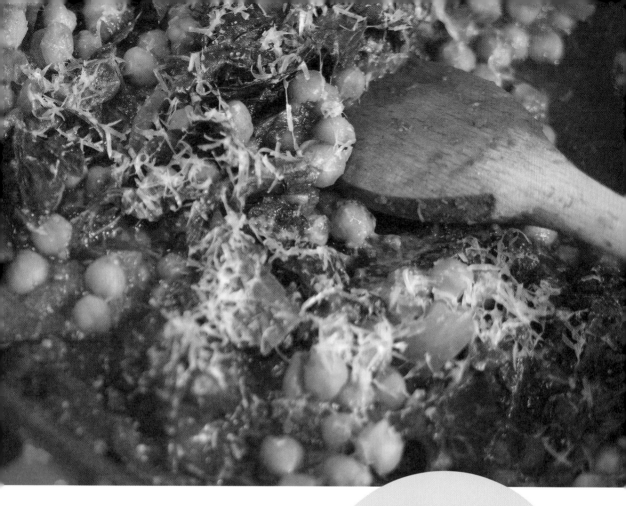

Heat the olive oil in a large, lidded saucepan over a medium heat. Add the onion and sauté, stirring frequently, until translucent. Add the garlic and ginger and cook for 1 minute, being careful not to burn them. Add the curry powder and stir, cooking for 1 minute. Then stir in the tomato paste and miso, cooking for a further minute.

Stir in the tomatoes, chickpeas and stock. Season to taste and cook over a low heat, half covered for 30–40 minutes. Add the silverbeet, cooking until it is just wilted. Transfer to 4 serving bowls and serve with parmesan (if using) and wholemeal bread.

Leafy greens

Silver beet, spinach and kale, are very nutritious. High in vitamins C and K, silver beet can promote a healthy heart, bones and skin. Along with other cruciferous vegetables it contains glucosinolates, which may help to protect against cancer.

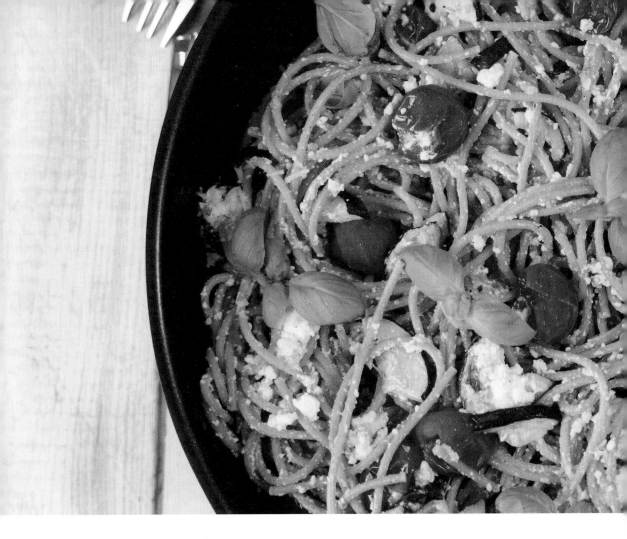

Spaghetti with zucchini, cherry tomatoes and ricotta sauce

SERVES 4

200 g (7 oz) cherry tomatoes

3 tablespoons extra virgin olive oil

2 small zucchini, halved lengthways and sliced

450 g (1¾ oz) wholemeal spaghetti

2 garlic cloves, chopped

200 g (7 oz) ricotta

80 g (2¾ oz) grated parmesan

zest of 1 lemon

½ lemon

1 cup basil leaves, loosely packed, to serve

salt and pepper to taste

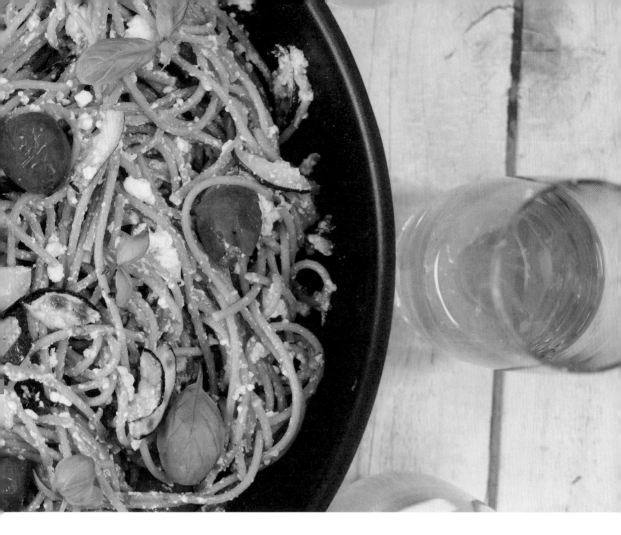

Preheat the oven to 220°C (430°F).

Place the cherry tomatoes on a baking sheet and season with salt, pepper and ½ tablespoon of olive oil. Roast until the cherry tomatoes are cooked and shrivelled but still holding their shape, about 5–10 minutes. Remove and set aside.

In the meantime, heat a large frying pan over a high heat and add the remaining oil. Working in batches, cook the zucchini until coloured but holding its shape. Once done, remove the zucchini from the pan and drain any remaining oil, leaving only 1 teaspoon. Set the pan aside.

Place a large pot of salted water over a high heat. Bring to a boil and cook the spaghetti according to the packet instructions. When the pasta is cooked, drain into a colander, reserving 1 cup of cooking liquid.

Meanwhile, when the spaghetti is nearly cooked, return the frying pan used for the zucchini to a low heat and add the garlic. Cook for 1 minute before adding the ricotta, parmesan, lemon zest and enough pasta cooking liquid to create a sauce. Season to taste and squeeze over the juice of half the lemon. Mix the zucchini, tomatoes and pasta through the sauce, mixing well. Serve topped with basil.

Soba noodles with shiitake and miso broth, tofu, mushrooms and kale

SERVES 4

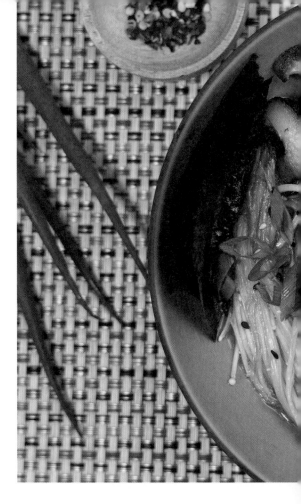

FOR THE BROTH

300 g (10½ oz) fresh shiitake mushrooms

5 French eschalots

1 carrot

1 tablespoon extra virgin olive oil

4 garlic cloves

6 thyme sprigs

50 g (1¾ oz) mirin

1.5 litres (51 fl oz) water

3 × 10 g (¼ oz) sachets organic powdered shiitake kombu dashi

4 dried shiitake mushrooms

2 tablespoons tamari

2 tablespoons red miso paste

½ knob fresh ginger, sliced

2 bay leaves

3 juniper berries

1 tablespoon black peppercorns

FOR THE SOUP

400 g (14 oz) mixed mushrooms (shiitake, enoki, shimeji, king oyster)

1½ tablespoons extra virgin olive oil

220 g (8 oz) Tuscan kale

300 g (10½ oz) organic teriyaki firm tofu, cubed

250 g (9 oz) soba noodles

2 cups coriander (cilantro) leaves, loosely packed

2 leaves roasted wakame seaweed, quartered

2 spring onions, sliced

2 tablespoons pickled ginger

2 tablespoons sesame seeds, roasted

salt to taste

To make the broth, finely slice the shiitake mushrooms, eschalots and carrot. Using a large, lidded pot over a high heat, warm 1 tablespoon of olive oil and add the sliced vegetables. Sauté until well coloured. Add the garlic, thyme and mirin. Keep cooking until almost all the released liquid has evaporated. Add the rest of the broth ingredients and simmer, covered, for 2 hours. Taste and adjust the flavour with more tamari or miso as needed. Strain the broth, removing the solids. Set aside the broth until ready to serve.

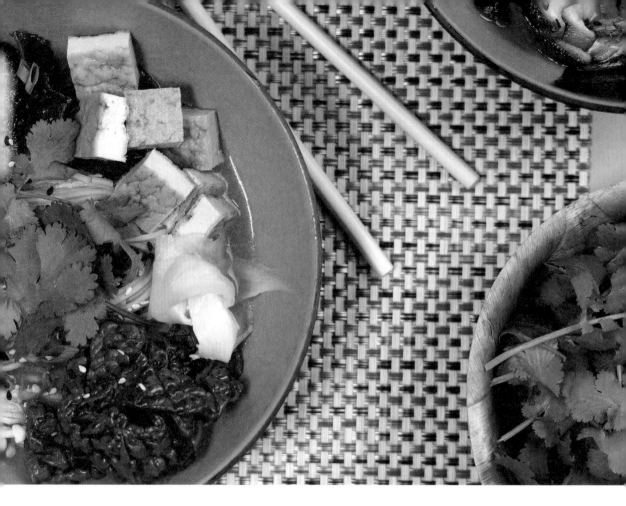

While the broth is cooking, prepare the toppings. Quarter the mushrooms and sauté in a hot pan with 1 tablespoon of olive oil until they start to colour. Cook in batches to avoid stewing the mushrooms. Set aside.

Remove the stem from the kale and cut the leaves into 7½ cm (3 in) pieces. Place in a bowl with ½ tablespoon extra virgin olive oil and mix to evenly coat. Place a frying pan on a high heat until extremely hot. Add the kale, only a few leaves at a time, and colour well on both sides. Repeat with the rest of the leaves. Lightly season with salt and set aside.

Place a large pot of salted water on a high heat and bring to a boil for the noodles. In the meantime, heat the tofu in a microwave and reheat the sautéed mushrooms and broth if they are no longer warm. Cook the soba noodles according to the packet instructions and refresh in cold water. Drain and divide amongst 4 serving bowls.

When ready to serve, top the noodles with the mushrooms, kale and tofu. Pour over hot broth and garnish with the remaining ingredients.

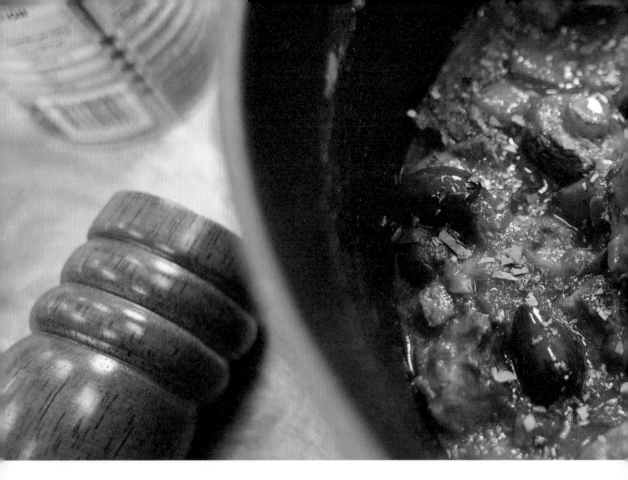

Seitan cacciatora

SERVES 4

¼ cup dried porcini mushrooms

3 tablespoons extra virgin olive oil

500 g (1 lb 2 oz) seitan (page 110), cubed

200 g (7 oz) button mushrooms

150 g (1¾ oz) onion, finely chopped

350 g (12½ oz) red capsicum, diced

4 garlic cloves, crushed

2 tablespoons tomato paste

2 × 400 g (14 oz) cans chopped tomatoes

350 ml (12 fl oz) vegetable stock

130 g (4½ oz) kalamata olives, pitted

30 g (1 oz) capers

2 teaspoons dried oregano

1 bay leaf

1 small rosemary sprig

salt and pepper to taste

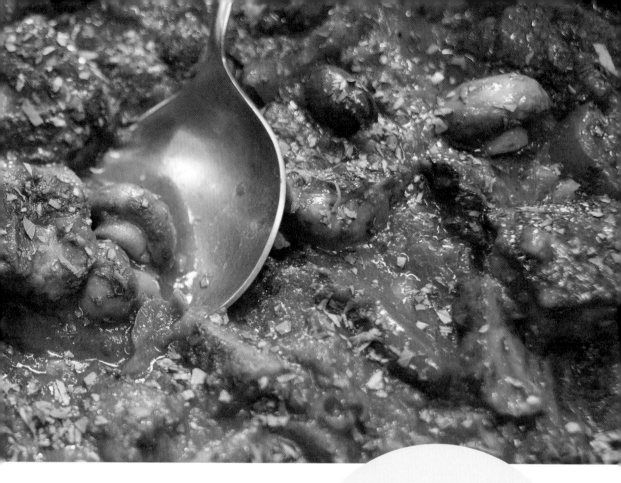

Place the dried porcini in a small bowl and just cover with boiling water. Let sit for 20 minutes.

In the meantime, place a heavy bottom frying pan over a high heat and add the olive oil. In batches, sauté the seitan cubes until well-coloured on all sides. Set aside.

Add the button mushrooms (halve any large ones) to the pan and colour well. Reduce the heat to medium and add the onion and capsicum, cooking until the onion is translucent. Add the garlic and cook for 1 minute. Add the tomato paste and cook for another minute, stirring well. Add the soaked porcini and all the remaining ingredients and mix well. Simmer, half covered, for 45 minutes, stirring occasionally. Add the seitan and stir through for a final 15 minutes.

Tofu

Tofu is a protein-rich food prepared by coagulating soy milk with lemon juice or calcium sulphate. 100 g of tofu contains 10 g of proteins packed in only 91 calories. Notably, the quality of soy protein is much higher than that of all the other beans and very similar to animal protein.

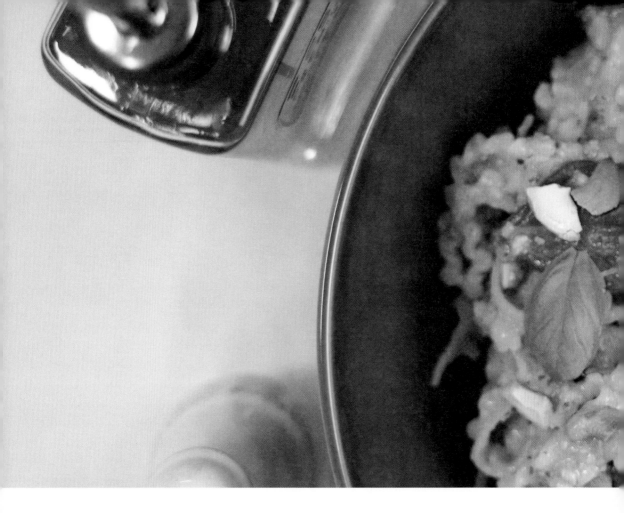

Ricciarelle with broad bean pesto and pecorino pepato

SERVES 4

250 g (9 oz) cooked broad beans (fresh or frozen)

1 garlic clove

70 g (2½ oz) raw cashews

50 g (1¾ oz) grated pecorino (plus extra to serve)

2 cups basil leaves (plus extra for garnish)

150 ml (5 fl oz) extra virgin olive oil

salt and pepper to taste

450 g (1¾ oz) ricciarelle or other long pasta

40 g (1½ oz) roasted cashews, roughly chopped

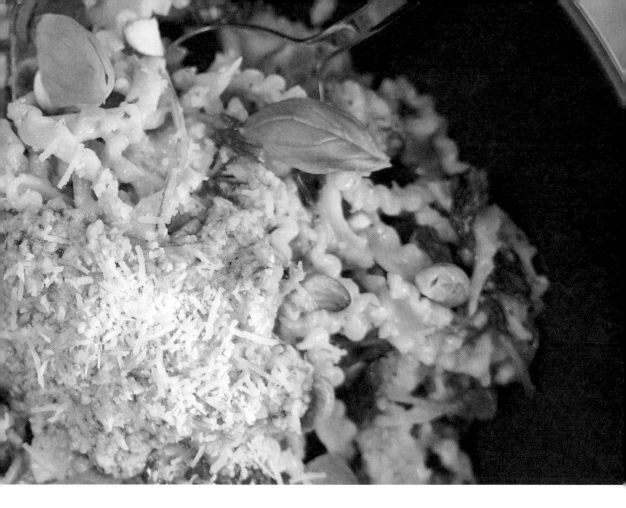

To make the pesto, place the broad beans, garlic, raw cashews, cheese and basil in a food processor and process until smooth. Add the olive oil and pulse until emulsified. Season to taste.

In the meantime, bring a large pot of salted water to the boil, and cook the pasta according to the packet instructions. Reserve 1 cup of the cooking liquid, then strain. Return the pasta to the pot, add the pesto and mix well, adding cooking water as needed to obtain a smooth and silky sauce.

Serve the pasta and top with extra basil leaves, cashews and pecorino.

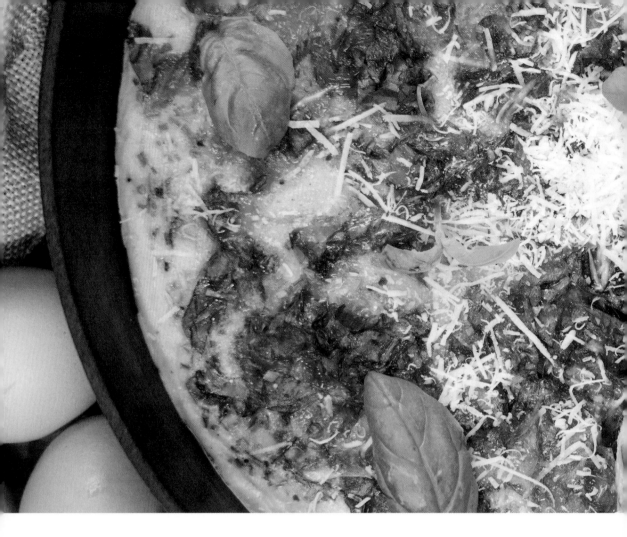

Rainbow chard frittata with purple sweet potato and pecorino

SERVES 4

1–2 medium purple sweet potatoes

10 large eggs

100 ml (3½ fl oz) skim milk

2 tablespoons chopped chives

150 g (1¾ oz) chard

2½ tablespoons extra virgin olive oil

50 g grated pecorino

½ cup basil leaves

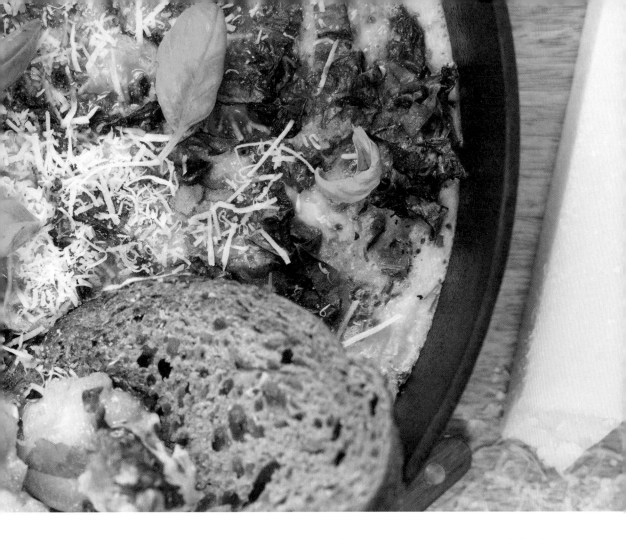

Preheat the oven to 200°C (400°F). Individually wrap the sweet potatoes in aluminium foil and place on a baking tray. Bake until tender (around 45–60 minutes). Remove from the oven and allow to cool. Once cool, peel the skins off and cut into 1 cm (½ in) slices. Lower the oven temperature to 180°C (350°F).

In a large bowl whisk the eggs, milk and chives. Season well and set aside. Strip the leaves from the chard stems and roughly chop. Finely chop the stems. Place a heavy-bottomed ovenproof pan over a medium heat and add 1 tablespoon of olive oil. Once hot add the chard stems and cook for 2 minutes until slightly soft. Add the leaves and wilt them slightly, seasoning well.

Transfer them to a bowl to cool slightly, then add to the egg mix. Stir well.

Wipe the inside of the pan and add the remaining olive oil. Return to the stovetop on high heat. Add the sweet potato and cook until some colour has developed. Pour over the egg and chard mixture and transfer the pan to the oven.

Bake until just set, about 7–14 minutes depending on the size of the pan, and top with pecorino and basil.

Orange vegetables

Eat carrots, pumpkins and sweet potatoes often. They are loaded with different carotenoids – responsible for their orange colour and for the production of vitamin A. This vitamin plays a key role in eye and immune-function health. In order to optimise carotenoid absorption and conversion to vitamin A, fat (for instance extra-virgin olive oil) needs to be eaten at the same meal as carrots, pumpkin or sweet potato.

Sweet potatoes contain the highest concentration of beta-carotene (31 mg in 100 g (3½ oz) of cooked vegetable), but pumpkin also provides generous amounts of alpha-carotene, zeaxanthin and lutein, making it a superior source of antioxidants.

Pumpkin's delicious, sweet flavour makes it a versatile ingredient for many recipes. Raw pumpkin can be added to a morning smoothie with fruits, avocado, nuts and dates or raisins. It can be roasted or baked, or used to prepare nutritious winter soups. Cooked pumpkin can be pureed with chickpeas, tahini, garlic and lemon juice for a colourful hummus.

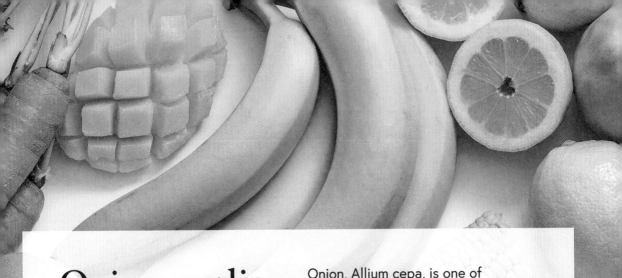

Onion, garlic and leeks

These vegetables are loaded with unique volatile organo-sulphur compounds, which give the vegetables their characteristic aroma and flavour. When garlic is cut or crushed, the compound alliin is exposed to alliinase, an enzyme that is essential to produce allicin. Allicin may lower the risk of heart disease by lowering blood pressure and cholesterol levels. Allicin can also be transformed into several bioactive compounds.

Onion, Allium cepa, is one of the richest sources of dietary flavonoids (fructooligosaccharides and thiosulfinates). Flavonoids, in particular, have shown to be important in the prevention of cardiovascular diseases and cancer. Red onions contain the highest levels of flavonols, while yellow onions contain only half as much.

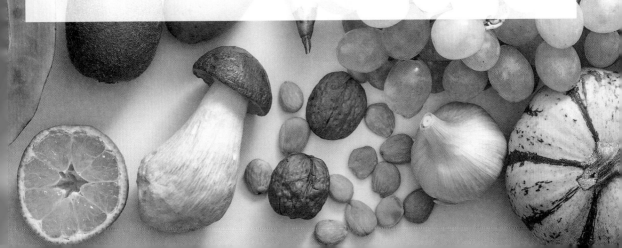

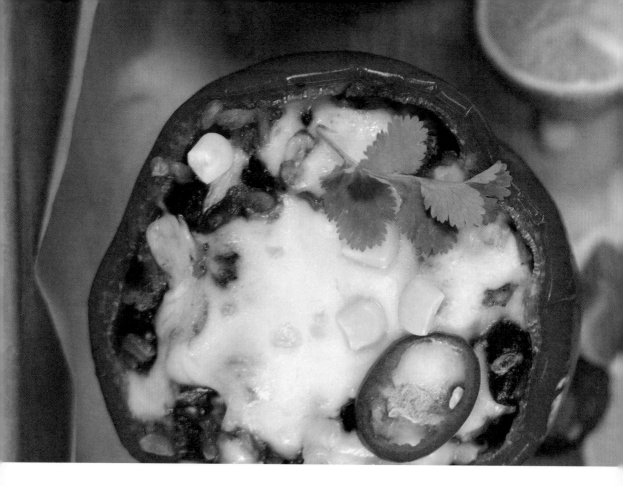

Mexican rice and bean-stuffed capsicums

SERVES 4

2 tablespoons extra virgin olive oil

1 small brown onion, finely diced

3 garlic cloves

½ teaspoon ground cumin

1 teaspoon ground coriander

1½ teaspoons smoked paprika

1 teaspoon dried oregano

¼ teaspoon chipotle powder

1 tablespoon thyme leaves

1½ tablespoons tomato paste

1 tablespoon chipotle peppers in adobo sauce, chopped

370 g (13 oz) brown rice

200 g (7 oz) canned chopped tomatoes

1.5 litres (51 fl oz) vegetable stock (plus extra if needed)

6 capsicums (3 red and 3 yellow)

180 g (6½ oz) cooked or canned sweet corn kernels

220 g (8 oz) cooked or canned black beans

25 kalamata olives, pitted and sliced

juice of 1 small lime

180 g (6½ oz) aged cheddar cheese, grated

1 cup coriander (cilantro) leaves, chopped

1 red chilli, sliced

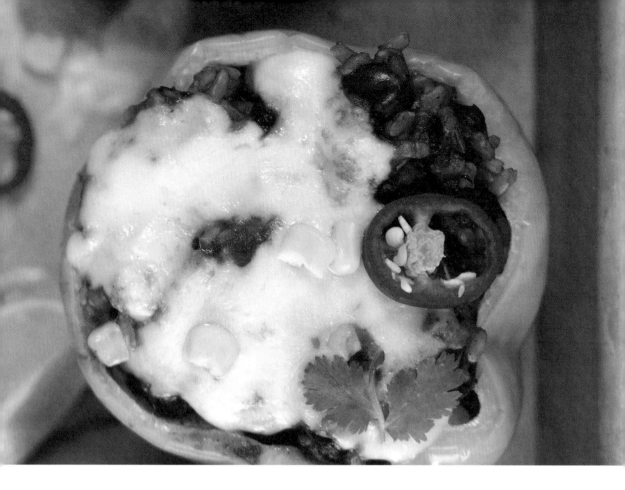

Preheat the oven to 180°C (350°F).

Heat the oil in a large pot over a medium heat. Add the onion and sauté until translucent. Add the garlic and cook, stirring, for 1 minute being careful not to burn it. Incorporate the spices and thyme and cook for another minute, stirring. Stir in the tomato paste and chipotle and cook for 1 minute. Add the rice, tomatoes and stock, season to taste and stir well. Cover with a lid and cook over a low heat until all the liquid has evaporated and the rice is cooked, about 30–40 minutes. Add extra stock if needed. Remove from the heat.

In the meantime, cut the tops off the capsicums and, keeping the capsicums whole, carefully remove the seeds. Stand them on a lined baking sheet and bake for 20 minutes. Remove and set aside.

Once the rice has cooled a little, stir in the corn, beans, olives, lime juice, half the cheese and half the coriander. Combine well and check for seasoning. Spoon the mix into the capsicums and top with the remaining cheese. Bake for 15 minutes or until heated through and the cheese has melted. Serve immediately, topped with sliced chilli and the remaining coriander.

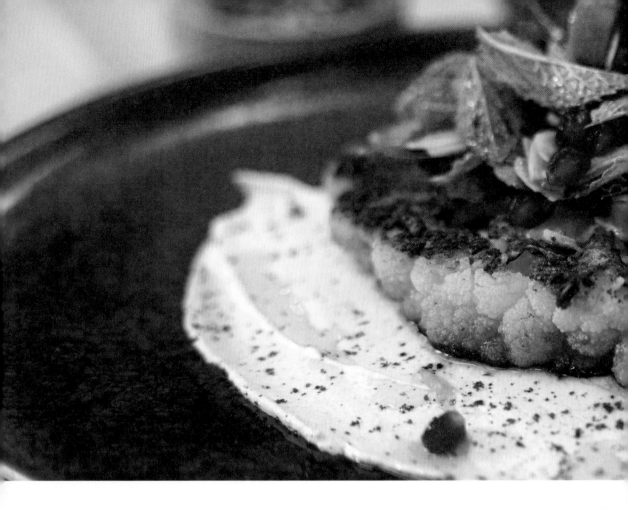

Cauliflower steaks with spiced labneh and pomegranate and herb salad

SERVES 4

2 medium cauliflowers

salt and pepper to taste

320 g (11½ oz) Labneh (page 184)

¼ teaspoon turmeric

¼ teaspoon ground cumin

¼ teaspoon ground coriander

1½ tablespoons lemon juice (plus extra for salad)

1½ tablespoons extra virgin olive oil

2 handfuls flat-leaf parsley, chopped

2 handfuls mint leaves

1 large pomegranate, deseeded

12 pitted green olives, sliced

2 tablespoons capers, drained

40 g (1½ oz) almond flakes, toasted

40 g (1½ oz) raisins

½ lemon

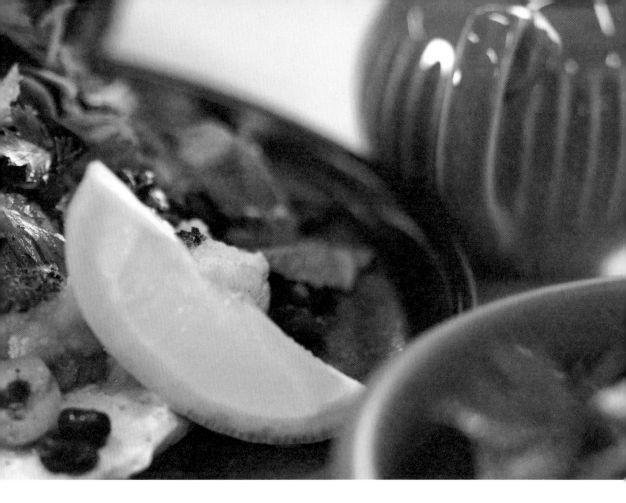

Preheat the oven to 180°C (350°F).

Hold the cauliflower heads firmly on a chopping board and cut 2 central slices (steaks), about 2½ cm (1 in) thick, from each. Be sure to include the core with each slice, to hold the florets together. The two outer cheeks will not be needed and can be used for another dish.

Heat a heavy-bottomed pan over a high heat. Working one piece at a time, place the cauliflower slices flat in the hot pan and colour them well on both sides.

Transfer the steaks to a lined baking sheet and season well with salt and pepper. Bake until cooked through (about 10 minutes).

In the meantime, prepare the labneh. Combine the labneh, spices and lemon juice in a bowl with 1 tablespoon of olive oil. Mix well and season with salt and pepper. Set aside.

In another bowl, combine the parsley, mint, pomegranate, olives, capers, almonds and raisins. Season with salt, a squeeze of lemon juice and olive oil. Mix well.

To serve, smear the labneh over 4 serving plates. Place the cauliflower steaks on top and scatter over the pomegranate and herb salad.

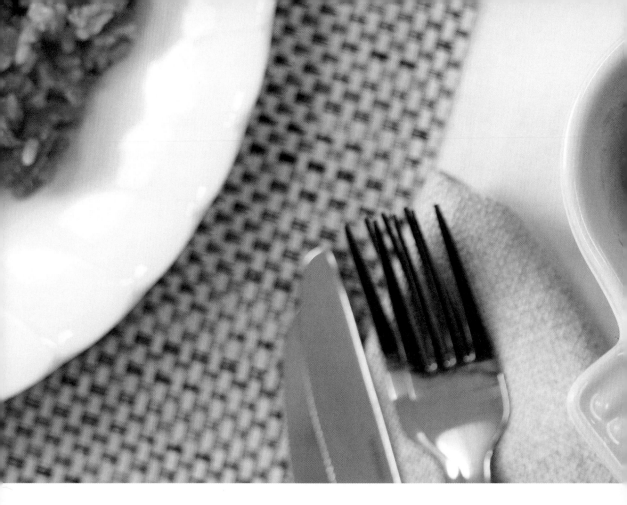

Brown rice and vegetable bake

SERVES 4

900 ml (30½ fl oz) vegetable stock

3 bay leaves

2 parmesan rinds (optional)

400 g (14 oz) brown rice

2 tablespoons extra virgin olive oil

1 small brown onion, finely diced

1 small yellow capsicum, finely diced

1 small red capsicum, finely diced

150 g (1¾ oz) button mushrooms, quartered

3 garlic cloves, minced

1 tablespoon tomato paste

1 tablespoon thyme leaves

2 teaspoons dried oregano

150 ml (5 fl oz) white wine

200 g (7 oz) canned chopped tomatoes

12 kalamata olives, pitted and halved

12 green olives, pitted and halved

1 tablespoon capers, drained

5 preserved artichokes, quartered

130 g (4½ oz) cooked chickpeas

3 cups baby spinach, loosely packed

salt and pepper to taste

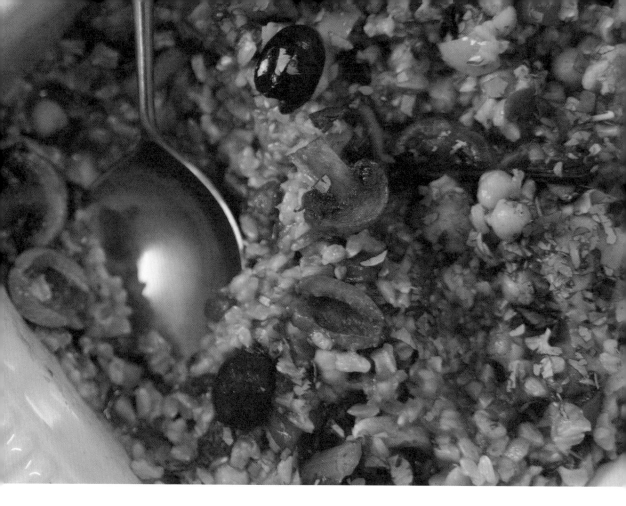

Preheat the oven to 170°C (340°F). Place a casserole dish in the oven to heat.

In a large saucepan over a high heat, place the stock, bay leaves and parmesan rind (if using). Bring to a boil. Once the casserole dish is hot and the stock has come to a boil, carefully add the rice and stock to the casserole, stir well, then half cover with a lid or foil and bake for 30 minutes.

In the meantime, rinse and dry the saucepan and return it to the heat with the olive oil, onion, capsicum and mushrooms. Sauté while stirring until the onion is translucent, add the garlic and cook for a further minute. Add the tomato paste, thyme, oregano and wine. Cook until the wine has evaporated, then remove from the heat and set aside.

Remove the casserole dish from the oven after 30 minutes. Add the vegetable mixture and mix well, together with the remaining ingredients except the spinach leaves. Return to the oven half covered and bake until the rice is done (about 15–20 minutes) and almost all the moisture has evaporated. Add more stock if required.

Remove from the oven, discard the bay leaves, and stir through the spinach until just wilted. Check for seasoning and serve.

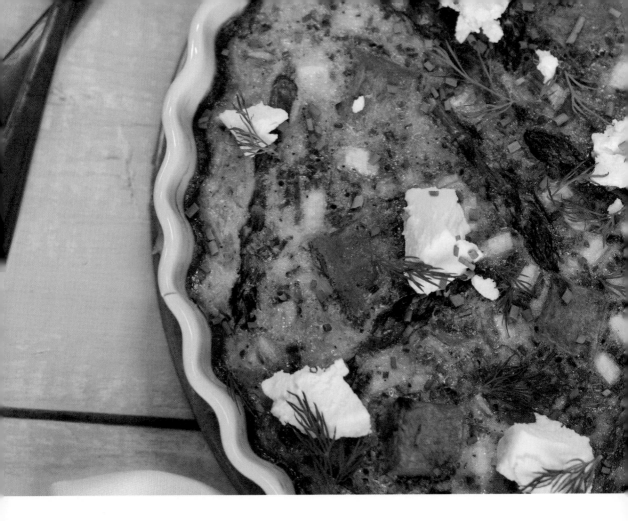

Asparagus, pumpkin frittata with herbs and goat's curd

SERVES 4

250 g (9 oz) pumpkin, peeled and cut into 2½ cm (1 in) dice

1½ tablespoons extra virgin olive oil (plus extra for brushing)

10 asparagus spears

10 large eggs

100 ml (3½ fl oz) skim milk

1 tablespoon chopped dill

1 tablespoon chopped chives

1 tablespoon chopped tarragon

60 g (2 oz) goat's curd or cheese

salt and pepper to taste

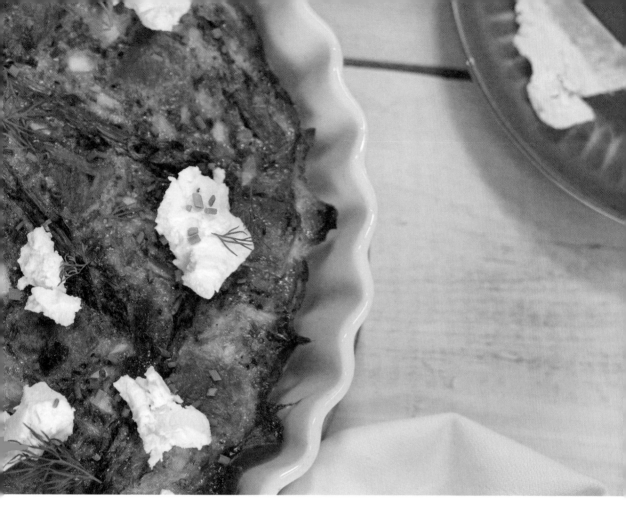

Preheat the oven to 180°C (350°F). Place the pumpkin on a lined baking sheet and season with salt, pepper and 1 tablespoon of olive oil. Bake for 15–20 minutes or until cooked through. Remove from the baking sheet and allow to cool.

Meanwhile, prepare the asparagus. Peel the lower half of each spear, then trim 1 cm (½ in) from the base and discard it. Place the asparagus on the baking sheet and season with salt, pepper and remaining ½ tablespoon of olive oil. Bake for 5–10 minutes or until the asparagus are just slightly undercooked. Remove from the heat. Once cool enough to handle, chop each asparagus stem into two or three pieces, leaving the tips whole.

Whisk the eggs and milk in a large bowl and season well. Stir through the herbs.

Brush the inside of a 25 cm (8½ in) pie dish with olive oil and place in the oven to preheat.

Pour the egg mix into the hot dish and distribute the pumpkin and asparagus evenly on top, pressing it in a little. Crumble the goat's cheese on top. Bake until just set, about 20–30 minutes depending on the size of the pan. Change from bottom to top heat as necessary to obtain desired colour and doneness. If necessary, finish cooking using the grill function to colour and set the top of the frittata.

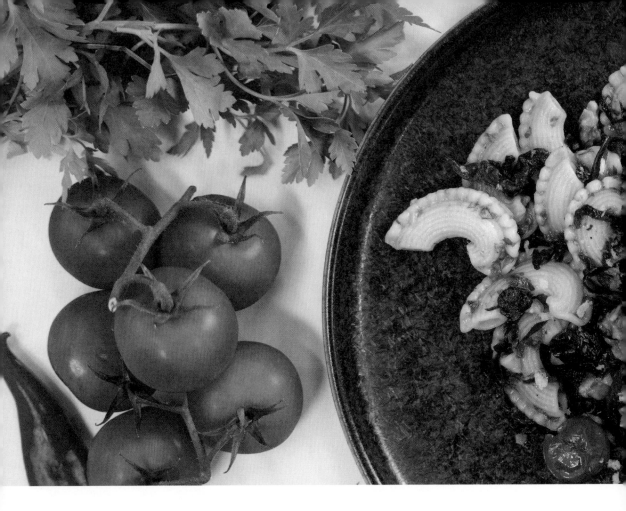

Creste di gallo with roasted cabbage, cherry tomatoes, garlic, chilli and walnuts

SERVES 4

200 g (7 oz) cherry tomatoes

3 tablespoons extra virgin olive oil

80 g (2¾ oz) panko breadcrumbs

40 g (1½ oz) grated parmesan

3 garlic cloves, minced

1 tablespoon chopped sage

zest of ½ lemon

200 g (7 oz) red cabbage, finely sliced

150 ml (5 fl oz) white wine

450 g (1¾ oz) creste di gallo pasta or other short pasta

60 g (2 oz) toasted walnuts, crushed

2 tablespoons chopped parsley

1 teaspoon dried chilli flakes

salt and pepper, to taste

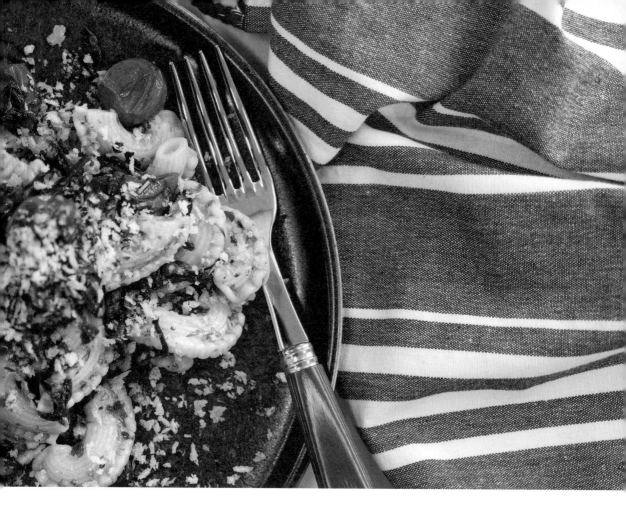

Preheat the oven to 140°C (285°F). Season the cherry tomatoes with salt, pepper and a dash of olive oil. Roast on a baking tray for 20–30 minutes, until shrivelled and softened but whole. Remove from the heat and set aside.

For the crumb, mix the panko crumbs, parmesan, 1 clove of garlic, sage and zest with 1½ tablespoons of olive oil. Add salt and pepper to taste. Transfer to a baking tray and cook, mixing several times, until evenly golden, about 7–10 minutes. Remove and set aside.

In the meantime, place a large pan over a high heat. Working in batches, sauté the cabbage in the remaining olive oil until well coloured and wilting. Return all the cabbage and the remaining garlic to the pan and cook until the garlic has a little colour but is not burnt. Season to taste and add the white wine, simmering until the liquid has almost completely evaporated. Remove from heat.

Bring a large pot of salted water to the boil, and cook the pasta according to the packet instructions. When the pasta is cooked, drain it, reserving 2–3 cups of pasta water. Return the pasta to the cooking pot, and toss through the tomatoes, cabbage, walnuts, parsley and chilli. Stir to combine. Add pasta water as needed to loosen the mixture and create a light sauce. Check for seasoning, serve immediately and top with the crumb.

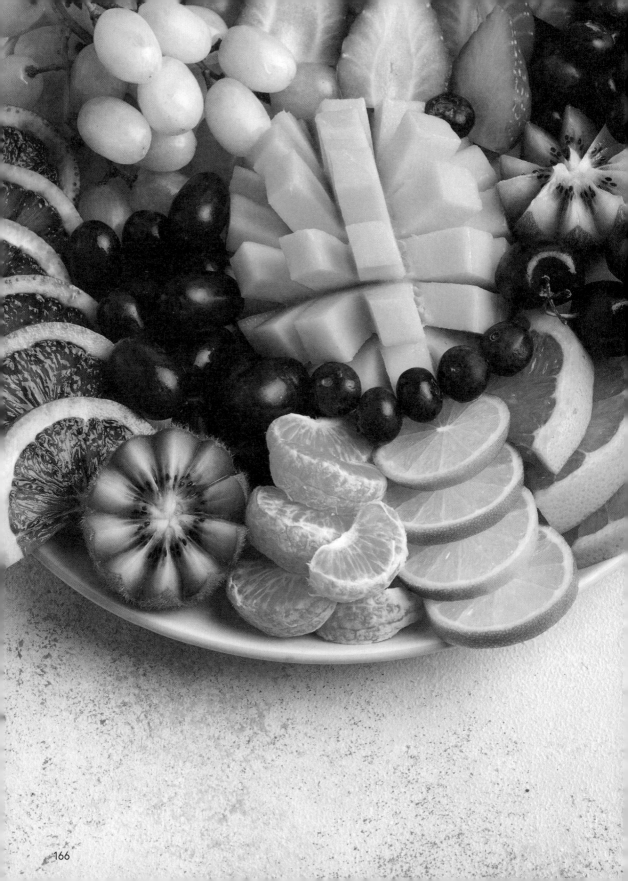

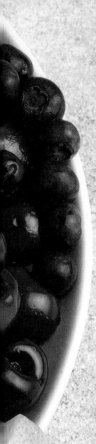

Desserts

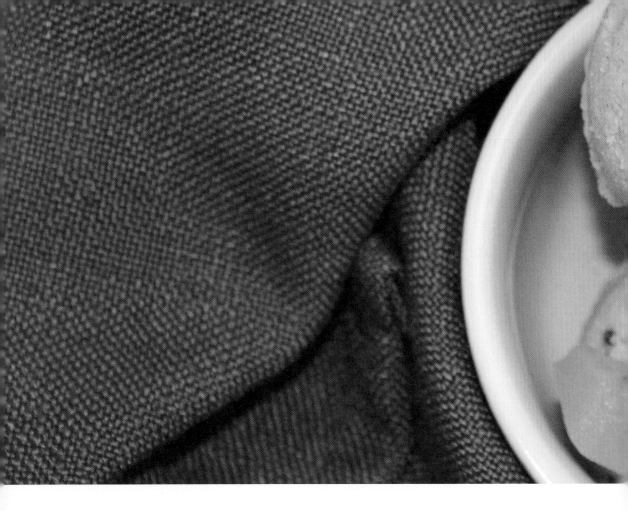

Vegan mango avocado passionfruit sorbet with pistachio

SERVES 4

1 medium avocado

300 g (10½ oz) mango flesh (fresh or frozen)

400 ml (13½ fl oz) can coconut cream (22% fat)

1 large banana, sliced

1 tablespoon flaxseed meal

30 g (1 oz) honey

3 passionfruit, pulp only

pistachios, crushed, to serve

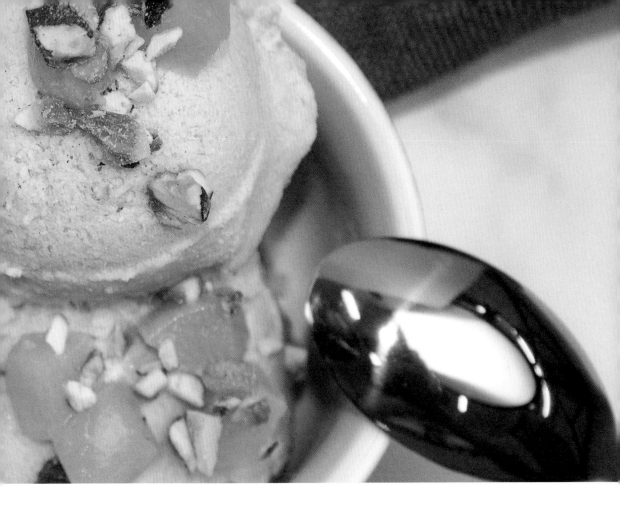

Cut the avocado in half and remove the stone. Spoon the flesh into a high-speed blender with all the remaining sorbet ingredients except the passionfruit. Blend well.

Place the passionfruit pulp in a small bowl and break it up well using a fork. Stir it through the blended mixture.

Using an ice-cream maker, process the mixture following the maker's instructions. Depending on the machine, you may need to strain and discard the passionfruit seeds. If you don't have an ice-cream maker, place the mixture in an airtight container in the freezer for 30 minutes. Remove from the freezer and mix well. Repeat every 30 minutes until almost frozen, then every 15 minutes until it is getting quite firm.

To serve, top scoops of sorbet with crushed pistachios.

Layered frozen fruit cake

SERVES 4

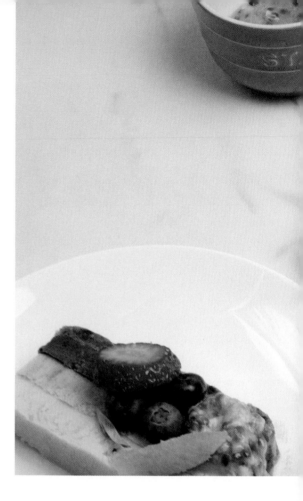

FOR THE BASE
50 g (1¾ oz) walnuts (soaked overnight and drained)

60 g (2 oz) raw cashews

45 g (1½ oz) cranberries

3 Medjool dates, pitted

FOR LAYER ONE
300 g (10½ oz) mixed berries

100 g (3½ oz) low-fat natural yoghurt

1 small banana

½ avocado

20 g (¾ oz) honey

2 Medjool dates, pitted

FOR LAYER TWO
150 g (1¾ oz) fresh pineapple, peeled, cored and diced

100 g (3½ oz) low-fat natural yoghurt

2 bananas

½ avocado

20 g (¾ oz) honey

2 Medjool dates, pitted

FOR LAYER THREE
200 g (7 oz) mango flesh (fresh or frozen)

1 small banana

120 g (4½ oz) low-fat natural yoghurt

½ avocado

50 g (1¾ oz) raw cashews

1 passionfruit

Lightly grease and line a rectangular loaf tin (12 cm × 25 cm) with baking paper. To prepare the base, pulse the walnuts and cashews in a food processor until coarsely ground. Add the cranberries and dates, and pulse again until the mixture starts clumping together. To check for the correct consistency, if you squeeze the mixture, it should be crumbly but will stick

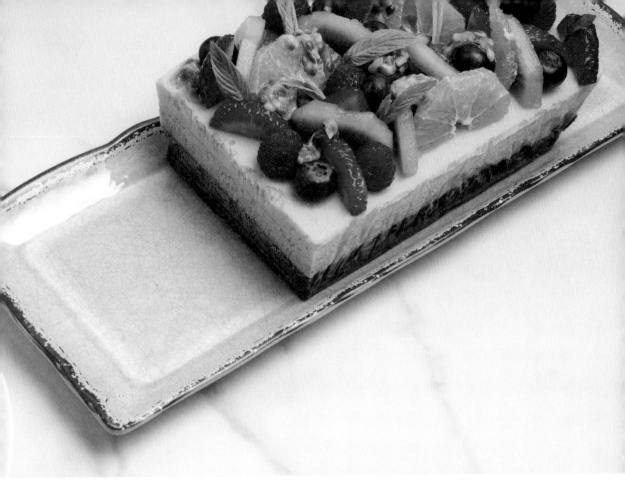

together. Spoon the mixture into the tin and press it firmly with the back of a spoon to create a flat layer. Freeze for about 1 hour.

In the meantime, make the three layers of filling. Blend the ingredients for each layer in a food processor, scraping down the blender if necessary to achieve a smooth puree. Pour each mixture into its own bowl, and chill in the fridge for about 1 hour.

Pour the first of the layers over the chilled base, then return the tin to the freezer for 1 hour or until the first fruit layer is starting to freeze. Then gently pour the second layer into the tin and return it to the freezer for 1 hour. If that layer is starting to freeze, pour over the final layer. Cover the tin with cling wrap and freeze

again, this time to set hard. Note: it's important to pour all three layers within the same period so they set at the same rate overnight.

When ready to serve, dip the lower half of the loaf tin carefully in hot water, or warm the base and sides of the tin with a hair drier, to loosen the sorbet. Invert the tin onto a serving plate to remove the sorbet, then slice it, using a knife dipped into hot water. Serve immediately.

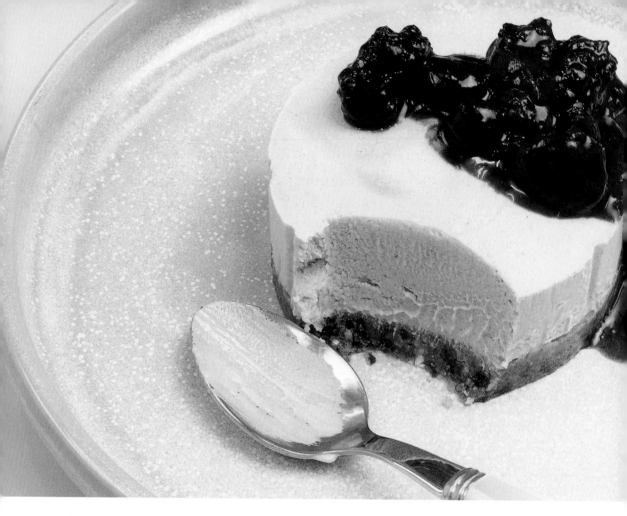

Vegan cheesecakes

MAKES 12

FOR THE BASE
50 g (1¾ oz) walnuts (soaked overnight and drained)

60 g (2 oz) raw cashews

45 g (1½ oz) cranberries

3 Medjool dates, pitted

45 g (1½ oz) raisins

50 g (1¾ oz) walnuts (soaked overnight and drained)

40 g (1½ oz) pine nuts

155 g (5½ oz) raw cashews (soaked overnight and drained)

320 ml (11 fl oz) almond milk

6 Medjool dates, pitted

juice of 4 lemons

zest of 1 lemon

½ avocado

½ teaspoon nutritional yeast

2 teaspoons vanilla essence

30 g (1 oz) honey

1 tablespoon extra virgin olive oil

TO SERVE
200 g (7 oz) raspberries or blueberries

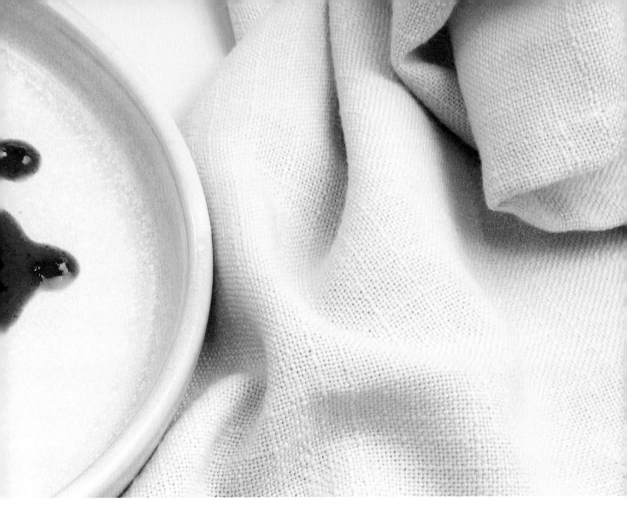

To prepare the base, pulse the walnuts and cashews in a food processor until coarsely ground. Add the cranberries and dates, and pulse again until the mixture starts clumping together. To check for the correct consistency, if you squeeze the mixture, it should be crumbly but will stick together.

Prepare a 12-cup muffin tray with a cupcake paper in each hole (or alternatively use greased rings or small round springform tins). Spoon 1 to 2 tablespoons of the crust mixture into each paper. Use your fingers or the base of a tumbler or the top of jar to press the base firmly down. If the mixture sticks to your fingers or the tumbler, wet them slightly. Once each

paper is filled, put the tray into the freezer to set for at least 30 minutes.

For the filling place all the filling ingredients in a high-speed blender and liquidise.

Divide the mixture amongst the frozen bases prepared earlier and return to the freezer.

When ready to serve, remove from the freezer and allow to thaw for 10–15 minutes. Top with fresh berries or poached fruit and enjoy.

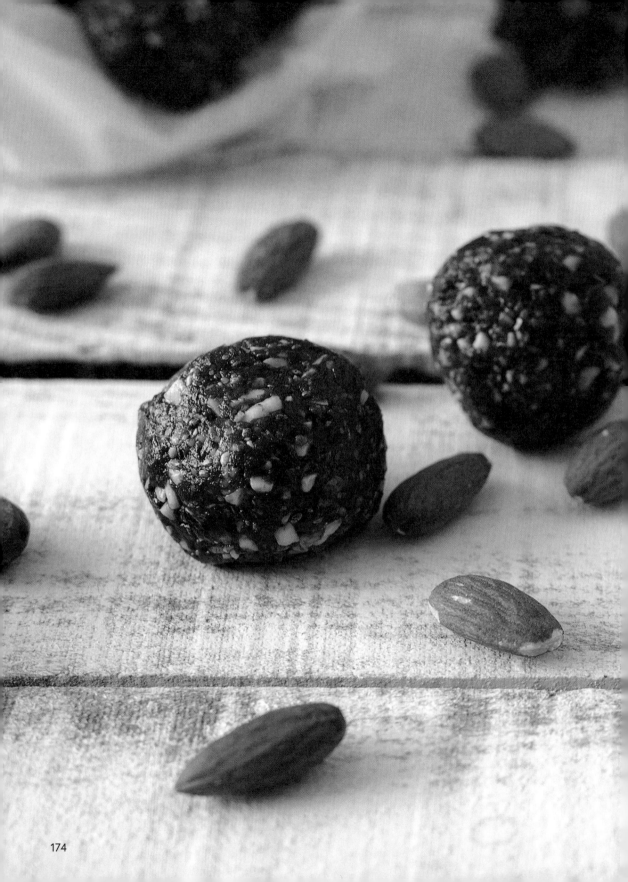

Sweet and savoury bites

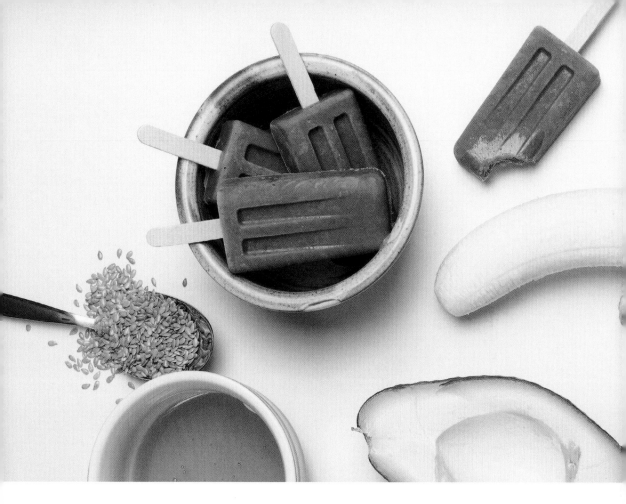

Avocado, banana and cacao popsicle

MAKES 4

400 ml (13½ fl oz) milk of choice

1 small ripe banana

½ ripe avocado

1 tablespoon flaxseeds (soaked overnight and drained)

2 tablespoons unsweetened cacao powder

30 g (1 oz) honey

3 Medjool dates, pitted

Put all the ingredients in a blender and process well until liquidised.

Pour the mixture into silicone popsicle moulds and insert the paddle sticks.

Place in the freezer until completely frozen and enjoy.

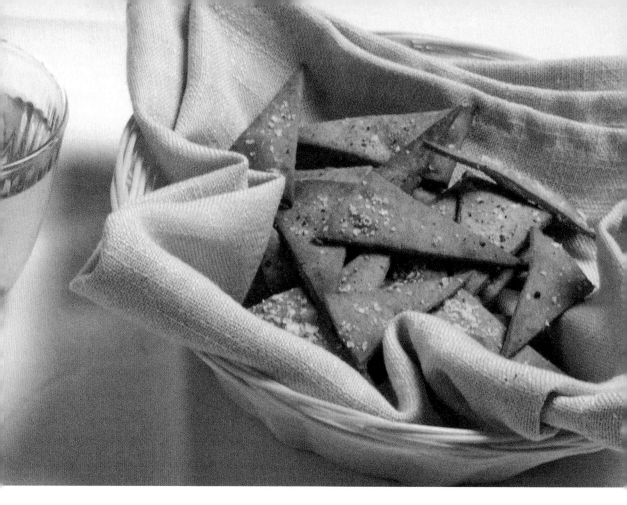

Buckwheat crispbread

MAKES 4

140 g (5 oz) buckwheat flour

100 g (3½ oz) almond meal

1 tablespoon flaxseed meal

½ teaspoon salt

2 tablespoons extra virgin olive oil

80 ml (2¾ fl oz) water

½ teaspoon dried rosemary

salt flakes and cracked black pepper

Preheat the oven to 180°C (350°F). To make the crispbread, place all the ingredients, except the salt and pepper, in a bowl and mix until a dough is formed. Knead lightly and divide into two.

Using a rolling pin, roll out each piece between 2 sheets of baking paper. Try to get an even thickness of 2 mm (⅛ in). Remove the top layer of baking paper and cut the dough into triangles. Working quickly before the surface dries, sprinkle with salt flakes and freshly cracked pepper. Bake for 7–12 minutes. Look for a rich brown colour. Cool on a rack, then store in an airtight container.

Nut and date energy bars

MAKES 16

FOR THE BARS
300 g (10½ oz) Medjool dates, pitted and chopped
180 g (6½ oz) dried apricots, chopped
90 g (3 oz) dried cranberries
90 g (3 oz) almonds, chopped
90 g (3 oz) cashews, chopped
45 g (1½ oz) pumpkin seeds
45 g (1½ oz) sunflower seeds
1 tablespoon peanut butter
6 tablespoons unsweetened cacao powder
50 g (1¾ oz) shredded coconut
1 teaspoon ground cinnamon

FOR THE TOPPING
40 g (1½ oz) peanut butter
20 g (¾ oz) honey
100 g (3½ oz) rolled oats
10 g (¼ oz) flaxseed meal
15 g (½ oz) coconut flakes, chopped
10 g (¼ oz) sesame seeds
pinch of salt
1 tablespoon water

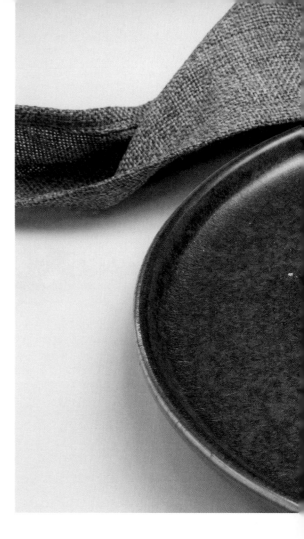

Preheat the oven to 160°C (320°F).

Place all the ingredients for the bar in a food processor and blend until they are finely chopped. Drizzle in some water, a little at a time, until the mixture starts coming together. It needs to be just firm. Turn the mixture out onto a lined 18 cm × 23 cm (7 in x 9 in) baking tray and spread into an even layer. Press the mix down with the back of a spoon and smooth the surface. Cover with cling wrap and set aside.

To make the topping, place all the ingredients in a bowl and mix thoroughly. Transfer to a lined baking sheet and cook for 20–30 minutes, mixing every five minutes, until well toasted.

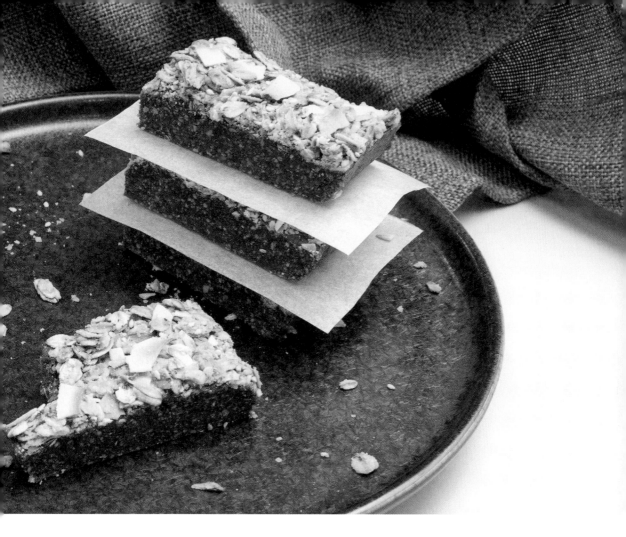

Remove from the oven and, without letting the topping cool, spoon it over the top of the bar, pressing down as before. Be careful, as the topping will still be hot. Place the bar in the fridge uncovered for at least 2 hours.

Carefully remove the chilled bar from the tray to a chopping board. Don't worry about any little bits crumbling. Cut into 16 squares. Wrap the squares individually in greaseproof paper to prevent them from sticking together, and store in an airtight container. The bars should keep for about a week.

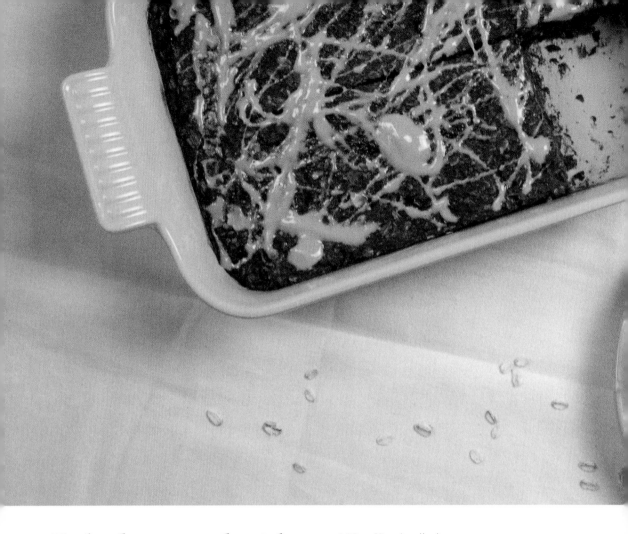

Baked oatmeal with cocoa, apple, banana and dried fruits

MAKES 20

360 g (2 oz) rolled oats

40 g (1½ oz) cocoa powder

1 pinch of salt

4 large very ripe bananas, mashed

100 g (3½ oz) peanut butter (plus extra to drizzle)

50 g (1¾ oz) date paste (see page 184)

2 eating apples

100 g (3½ oz) almonds, crushed

120 g (4½ oz) dried cranberries

120 ml (4 fl oz) almond milk

1 orange, juiced

1 orange, zest grated and segments chopped

peanut butter, to serve

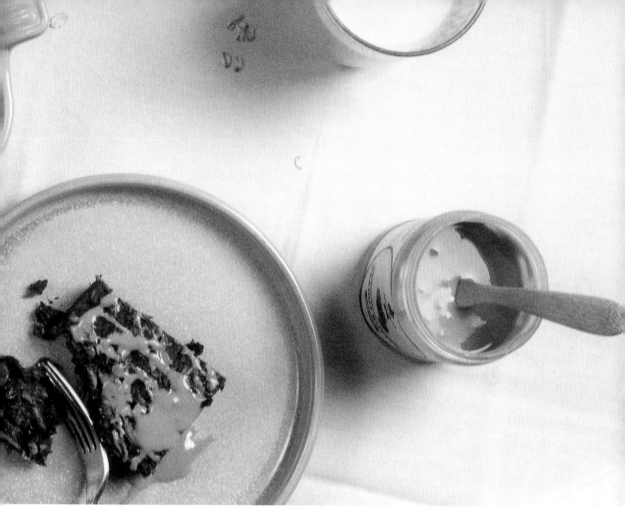

Preheat the oven to 180°C (350°F). Lightly grease a 20 cm × 30 cm (8 in × 12 in) baking tray or slice pan with baking paper.

Place the oats in a large bowl with the cocoa powder and salt. Mix well to ensure there are no cocoa lumps. In a separate bowl combine the mashed bananas, peanut butter and date paste, mixing thoroughly. Peel, core and dice the apples into 1 cm (½ in) pieces.

Add all the ingredients to the prepared oats and combine until it all binds well. Transfer the mixture to the baking tray and bake for 25–30 minutes until set. Cool slightly and cut into squares. Drizzle with a little softened and thinned peanut butter.

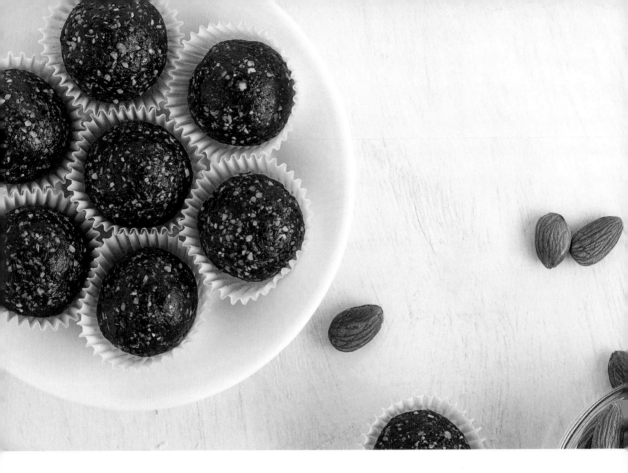

Date and hemp seed balls

MAKES 18

320 g (11½ oz) almonds (soaked overnight and drained)

80 g (2¾ oz) raisins

70 g (2½ oz) Medjool dates, pitted

40 g (1½ oz) desiccated coconut

70 g (1½ oz) hemp seeds

20 g (¾ oz) carob powder

½ teaspoon ground cinnamon

¼ teaspoon ground cardamom

Place all the ingredients in a food processor and blend until finely chopped. With the motor running, drizzle in some cold water, if needed, in order to achieve a soft dough texture.

Roll the mixture into small balls with your hands to the size that you prefer and enjoy. Will keep for a week in a sealed container, in the fridge.

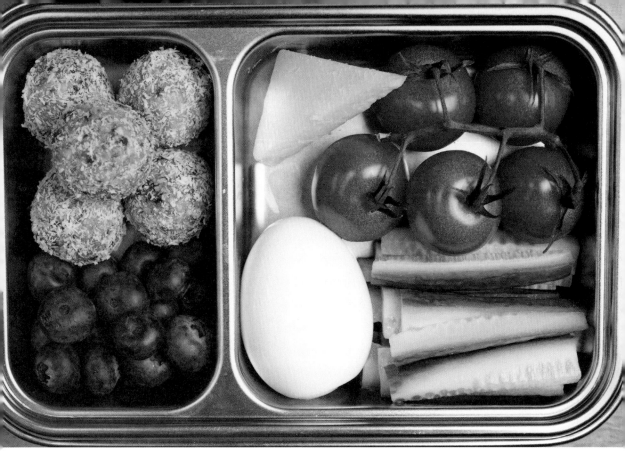

Mango and cashew balls

MAKES 12

140 g (1½ oz) dried mango

140 g (1½ oz) raw cashews

30 g (1 oz) goji berries

60 g (2 oz) desiccated coconut (plus extra for coating)

½ teaspoon turmeric powder

zest of 1 lemon

Place all the ingredients in a food processor and blend until finely chopped. With the motor running, drizzle in some cold water a little at a time until the mixture starts to come together. Roll the mixture into small balls with your hands and roll in desiccated coconut. Store in an airtight jar.

Date paste

MAKES ¾ CUP

200 g (7 oz) Medjool dates, pitted

Place the dates in a small heatproof bowl, and pour over enough boiling water to just cover them. Cover and allow the dates to sit for a minimum of 4 hours, but ideally overnight.

Strain the dates and reserve the liquid. Place the dates in a blender and process to a fine paste, adding some of the reserved liquid if necessary. Make sure the dates are blended evenly. Transfer to a sealed container and store in the fridge for up to 4 weeks.

Lavosh

3 nori seaweed sheets (optional)
180 g (6½ oz) wholemeal flour
100 g (3½ oz) rye flour
7 g (¼ oz) salt
7 g (¼ oz) baker's yeast
160 ml (5½ fl oz) warm water
30 ml (1 fl oz) extra virgin olive oil
1 tablespoon black sesame seeds
1 tablespoon white sesame seeds

To make the nori powder (if using) place the nori sheets in a high-speed blender and blend to a fine powder. Place the flours, salt and nori in the bowl of a stand mixer. In a separate bowl mix the yeast, water and oil. Start the mixer on a low setting with the hook attachment. Slowly pour in the yeast mixture and keep mixing until a velvety dough is formed. Cover with

cling wrap and refrigerate for 2–12 hours. Once rested, preheat the oven to 170°C (340°F).

Cut the dough into pieces about the size of a small lemon, and roll out on a lightly floured surface (or use a pasta machine) until 2 mm (⅛ in) thick. Top with the sesame seeds and bake on a lined baking sheet until golden and crispy. Lavosh can be stored in a sealed tin for a week or two.

Guacamole

2 ripe avocados
2 tablespoons onion, finely diced
2 tablespoons fresh lime juice
½ garlic clove, finely chopped
1 tablespoon coriander leaves, finely chopped
½ tablespoon extra virgin olive oil
salt and pepper to taste

For the guacamole, place the avocado flesh in a bowl and mash with a fork. Fold through the remaining ingredients, transfer to a serving bowl, cover and place in the fridge. Serve on the same day.

Labneh

500 g (1 lb 2 oz) full-fat sheep's yoghurt

The night before you want to use the labneh, place the sheep's yoghurt into a cheesecloth-lined colander over a mixing bowl. Leave it to drain overnight. Discard the drained whey, transfer the labneh to a bowl and refrigerate. Store for 3–4 days.

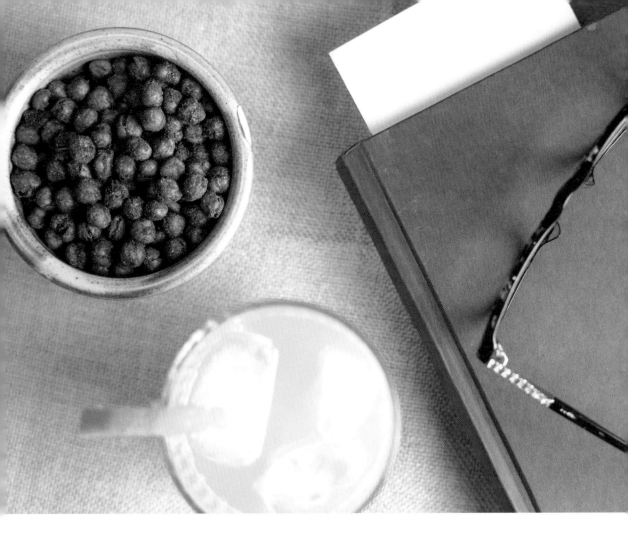

Crispy spiced chickpeas

450 g (1¾ oz) canned chickpeas

30 ml (1 fl oz) extra virgin olive oil

1½ teaspoons Madras curry powder

1½ teaspoons smoked paprika

1½ teaspoons nutritional yeast

½ teaspoon smoked chipotle powder

½ teaspoon fine salt

1 pinch ground pepper

Rinse the chickpeas thoroughly in a colander until the water runs clear. Drain well. Spread the chickpeas out on a clean towel, and rub thoroughly to dry them off as much as possible. Discard any skins that fall off. Place the chickpeas on a lined baking sheet and refrigerate uncovered for 4–12 hours to further dry them.

Preheat the oven to 220°C (430°F). In a bowl, toss the chickpeas with the remaining ingredients and mix well. Transfer to a large, lined baking tray. Bake for 20 minutes, then lower the temperature to 160°C (320°F). Cook for a further 40–60 minutes; be careful not to burn the spices. Cool before serving. Store in a tightly sealed jar in the pantry for up to a week.

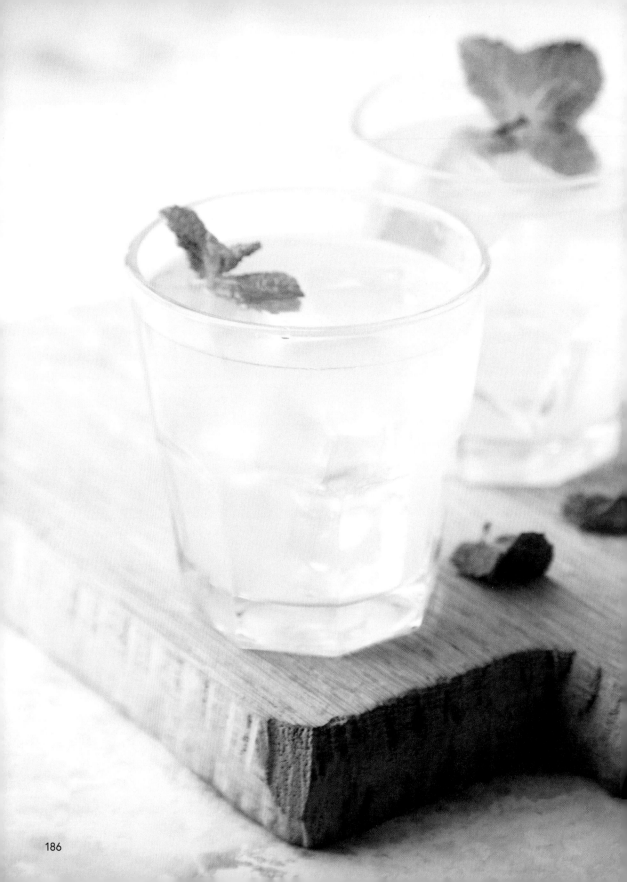

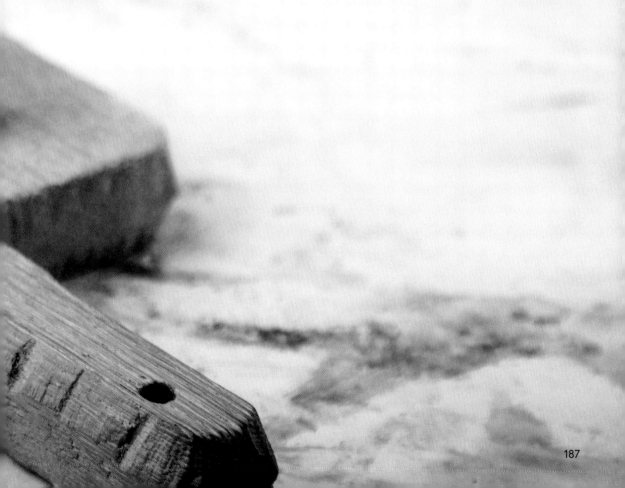

Smoothies, teas and drinks

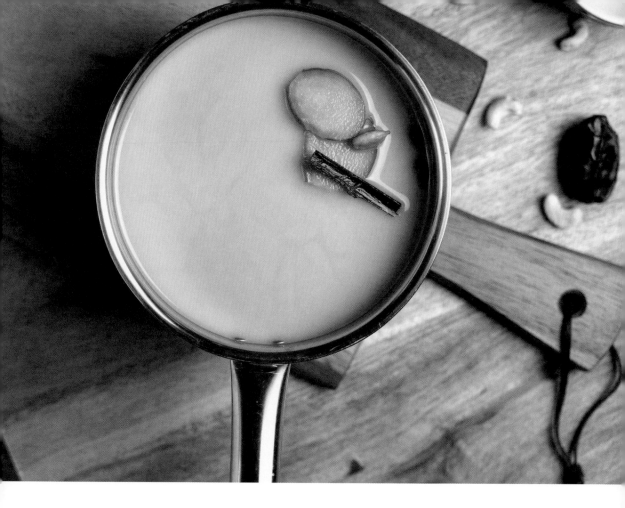

Homemade chai with cashew milk

SERVES 4

200 g (7 oz) raw cashews

1 litre (34 fl oz) water

½ tablespoon fennel seeds

3 cardamom pods

6 whole cloves

1 star anise

3 black peppercorns

1 cinnamon stick

1 knob fresh ginger, thinly sliced

1 tablespoon Darjeeling tea leaves

Date paste (page 184) to taste

For the cashew milk, place cashews and water in a high-speed blender and blend for 1–2 minutes. Strain through a piece of cheesecloth into a medium saucepan.

Add the spices and ginger to the cashew milk and stir well. Bring to a boil over high heat, then reduce to a simmer for 5–7 minutes.

Remove pan from the heat and stir through the tea leaves. Set aside to steep for 10 minutes, then strain. Return the strained chai to the saucepan. Reheat and sweeten with date paste to taste. Serve immediately.

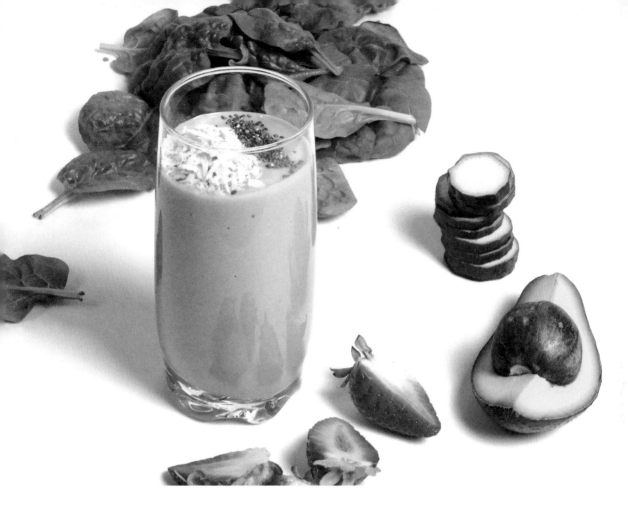

Strawberry, zucchini and avocado smoothie

SERVES 4

1 cup fresh strawberries, hulled

½ zucchini (courgette), diced

1 small avocado, flesh diced

¼ cup baby spinach

1 cup ice cubes

125 ml (4 fl oz) almond milk, unsweetened

½ orange, juiced

1 teaspoon fresh ginger, grated

1 tablespoon honey

Place all the ingredients, except the honey, in a high-powered blender and blend at high speed for 1 minute. Add the honey and keep blending until smooth.

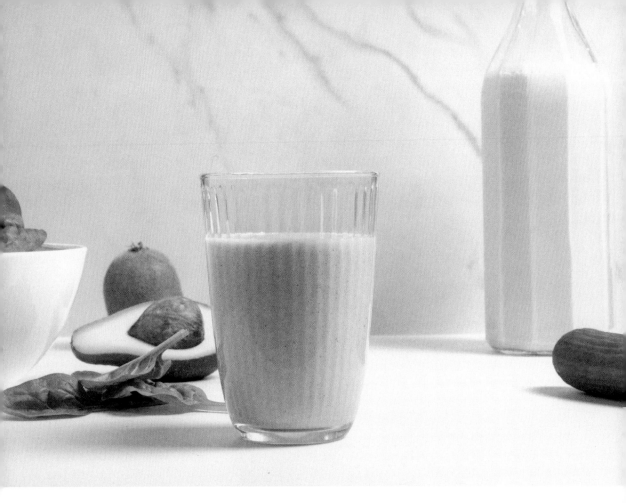

Cucumber, kiwi and avocado smoothie

SERVES 4

1 large cucumber, sliced

1 kiwifruit, peeled and diced

1 small avocado, flesh diced

1 green apple, peeled, cored and diced

¼ cup spinach

1 cup ice

¾ cup almond milk, unsweetened

1 tablespoon almond butter

1 tablespoon honey

Place all ingredients, except the honey, in the blender and blend at high speed for 1 minute. Add the honey and keep blending until smooth.

Pour into four glasses and enjoy.

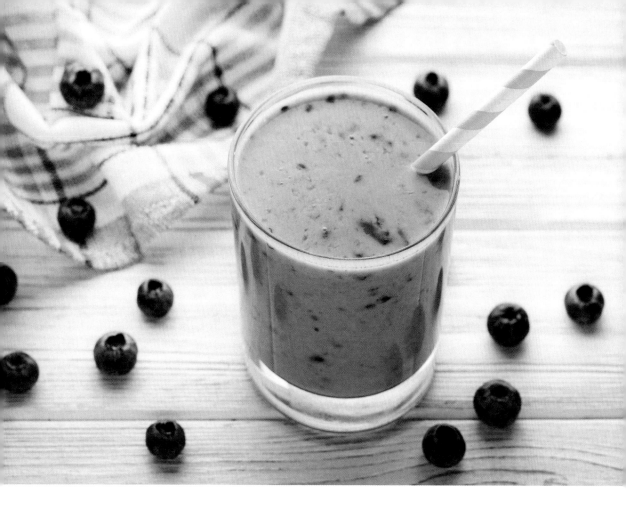

Blueberry and lavender lassi

SERVES 4

180 g (6½ oz) blueberries
350 g (12½ oz) low-fat natural yoghurt
1½ tablespoons honey
350 ml (12 fl oz) water
2 teaspoons dried lavender

Place the blueberries, yoghurt, honey and water in a high-speed blender and liquidise.

Pour into an airtight container and stir in the dried lavender. Rest in the fridge overnight.

The next day, strain and discard the lavender. Then it is ready to serve.

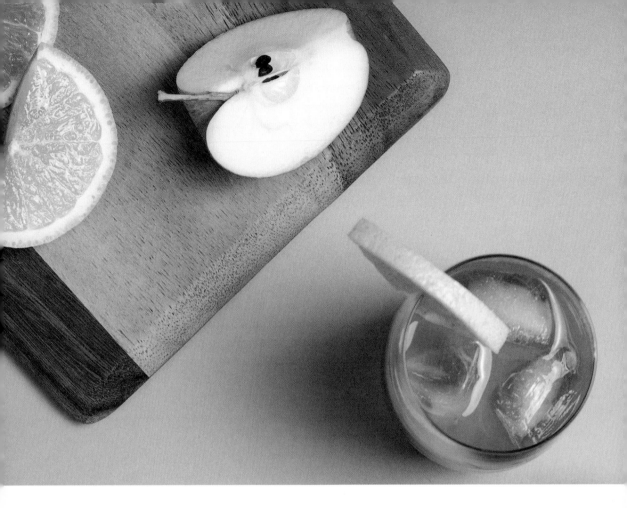

Rhubarb, apple and ginger juice

SERVES 4

300 g (10½ oz) rhubarb stems, trimmed

3 eating apples (royal gala or pink lady), peeled and cored

2 oranges, juiced

125 ml (4 fl oz) water

20 g (¾ oz) fresh ginger, grated

1 tablespoon honey

Place all the ingredients, except the honey, in a blender and blend at high speed for 1 minute. Add the honey and keep blending until well liquidised. Strain through a piece of cheesecloth or a very fine mesh strainer.

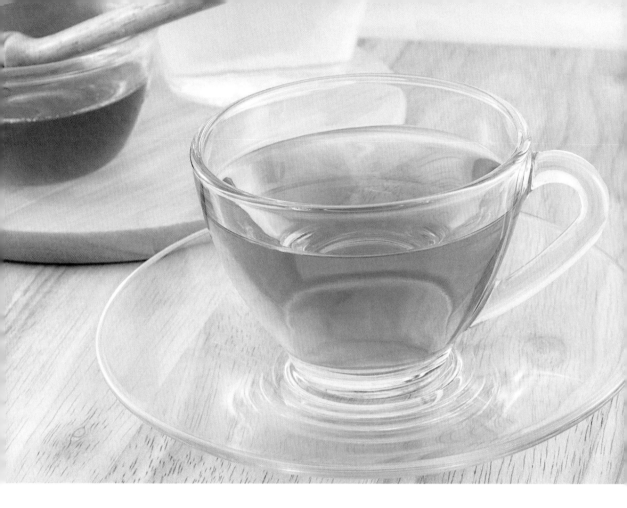

Refreshing tea

SERVES 2

MINT TEA
1 large sprig of fresh organic mint (extra for
  serving)

honey to taste

Place the mint in a 2 cup teapot and pour over
freshly boiled hot water. Leave to steep for
20 minutes. Strain into a cup and add honey
and extra fresh mint leaves if desired.

To serve chilled set aside to cool and add
icecubes to serve.

COCOA NIB TEA
20 g (¾ oz) cocoa nibs

honey to taste

nut milk, if desired

Place the cocoa nibs in a 2 cup teapot and pour
over freshly boiled hot water. Leave to steep
for 20 minutes. Strain into a cup. Add honey
to taste and a splash of nut milk if desired.

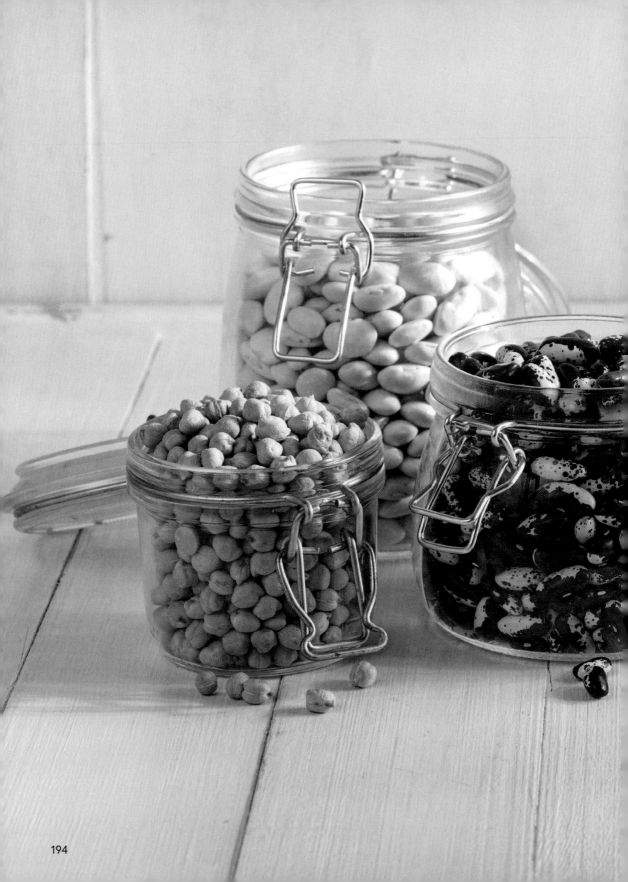

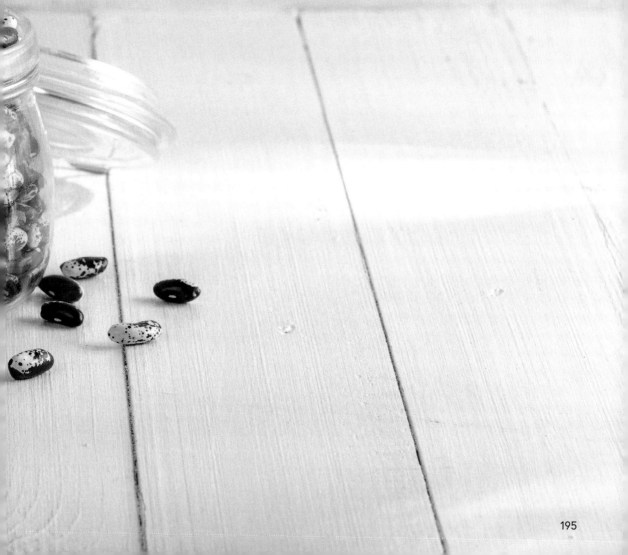

Whole grains and legumes

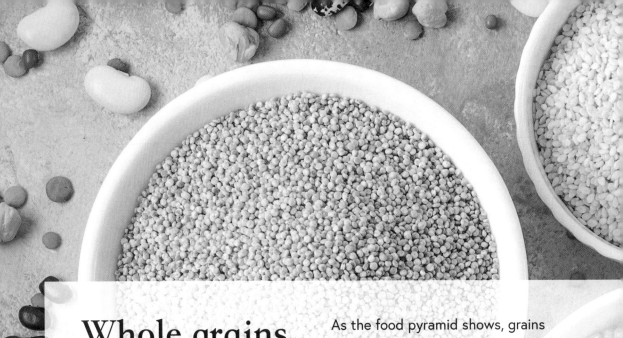

Whole grains and legumes

Wheat, barley and legumes rather than meat were the staple food of gladiators in Ancient Rome, as a study on their bones by the Department of Forensic Medicine at the Medical University of Vienna has demonstrated.

As the food pyramid shows, grains and beans should be consumed daily. Unlike refined carbohydrates, the consumption of minimally processed whole grains and beans are essential for optimal health.

A combination of legumes and whole grains also provides all the essential amino acids, important to form all proteins in our body, without atherogenic fatty acids promoting plaque build-up inside the

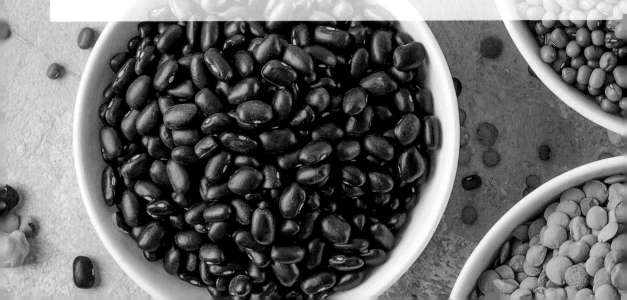

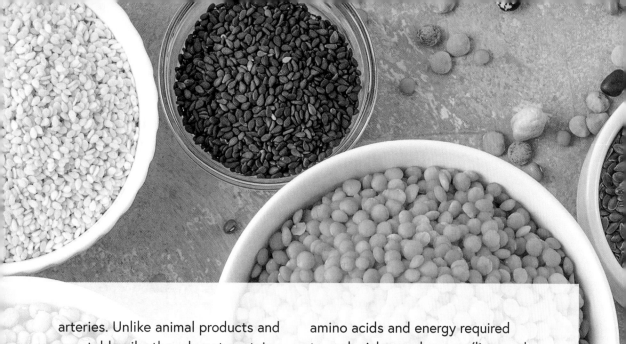

arteries. Unlike animal products and vegetable oils, they do not contain any saturated or trans-fatty acids, or other unhealthy ingredients.

However they do contain many calories; this is why we need to consume the right amount of them, based on our physiological needs. If we perform lots of manual work, or exercise hard, we need to eat higher amounts of whole grains and legumes to provide the essential amino acids and energy required to replenish our glycogen (liver and muscle concentrated glucose) stores in the liver and skeletal muscle. If we are sedentary, we need to eat less. But the higher the consumption of minimally processed whole grains and beans, the higher the intake of a variety of protective vitamins, minerals, phytochemicals and dietary fibres as well.

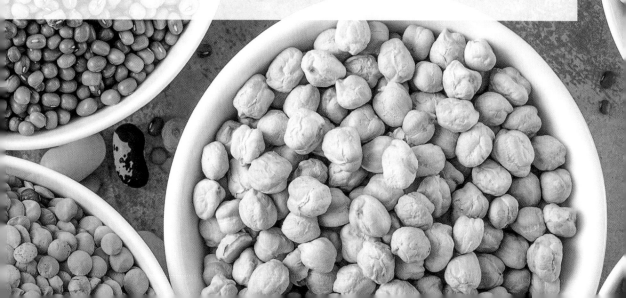

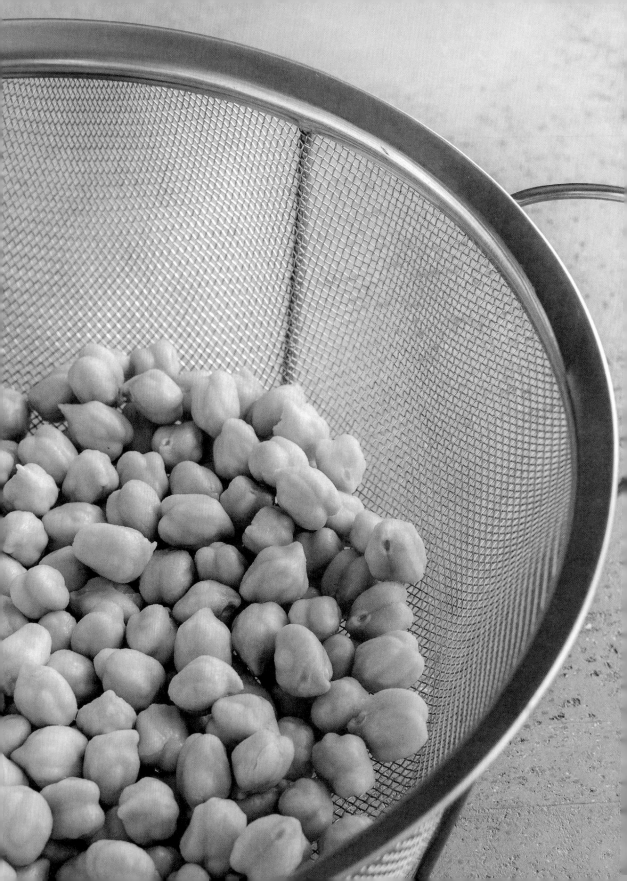

The magic of meal prep: whole grains & beans ready to go!

Stocking your pantry with a variety of whole grains and legumes is practical and essential for a nutritious diet. When stored properly in a cool, dark place, these staples can last for months, providing a reliable base for countless meals. Contrary to common misconceptions, preparing legumes and whole grains is simple and can significantly boost your nutritional intake.

When dealing with dried legumes, soaking is crucial and can be done in two ways:

1. Long Soak: Rinse the legumes thoroughly, then immerse them in warm water using a container with five parts water to one part legumes. Soak them overnight, discarding any that float in the morning and rinsing the rest.

2. Quick Soak: After a thorough rinse, place the legumes in a pot with water five to six times their volume. Bring to a boil, cook for a couple of minutes, then turn off the heat and let them rest for three to four hours.

Soaking reduces phytic acid, which inhibits mineral absorption. Adding a tablespoon of lemon juice or apple cider vinegar per litre of water enhances this process. Studies show soaking can cut phytic acid in beans from 2.99 mg/100 g to 1.64 mg/100 g.

The next step, which improves digestibility, is cooking. Adding herbs like bay leaves or rosemary can help. Cooking reduces trypsin inhibitors in legumes by 80 – 90 per cent, improving protein digestion. Studies show that cooking boosts protein assimilation, especially in chickpeas, increasing from 55 per cent to 94.9 per cent.

Simmer legumes gently for one to two hours, depending on the type, until tender. Use plenty of water, as they absorb a lot during cooking. Skim off any foam and, once cooled, season lightly with salt. Store in glass containers in the refrigerator to keep them fresh for various dishes throughout the week.

This method also works for whole grains like brown rice, farro and barley. Cooking these grains in advance ensures you always have a healthy base for meals. Pre-cooked grains and legumes can be added to salads, soups, or used as a side dish. For a quick, nutritious salad, mix cooked legumes or grains with fresh vegetables and dress with lemon juice, extra-virgin olive oil and a touch of balsamic vinegar to enhance nutrient absorption.

By dedicating a small amount of time each week to preparing these basics, you'll find it easier to create balanced, nutritious meals, even on busy days. This habit not only simplifies your cooking routine but also ensures you and your family consistently enjoy wholesome, homemade meals rich in the benefits of whole grains and legumes. Regularly incorporating these nutrient-dense foods into your diet can improve overall health, providing the energy and nutrients needed to thrive.

Home cooked beans and legumes

There is a misconception that legumes and whole grains are hard to prepare. That is completely wrong. They're a great product to keep in your pantry.

The easiest way to make sure you have them ready to add to meals is to prepare them once or twice a week – two or more different varieties is a good idea – and store them in the fridge until you need them.

Large beans, such as chickpeas and fava and borlotti beans, should be soaked for 24 hours before cooking.

Whenever you're cooking, you can add a cup or two of dried beans, chickpeas or lentils to a saucepan and simmer them until done. Use at least three cups of water for every cup of beans since they are nature's little sponges. Keep an eye on water levels as they're cooking and skim off any foam that rises.

Drain the beans and, once cooled, add a little salt and store them in the fridge ready for use. This also works for grains like brown rice, farro and barley. These cooked grains and legumes can easily be added to salads and soups at meal times. If you're using them in salads, a bit of lemon juice improves the taste and the availability of vitamins and minerals, especially calcium and iron.

BEANS AND LEGUMES

Always have a variety of wholegrains and legumes in your cupboard. Unlike many other food products, they will last for several months stored at room temperature and in dark conditions.

To keep a steady supply of beans, lentils or chickpeas on hand, cover a cup of your choice of legume with plenty of water and set it aside to soak overnight. Soaking reduces the production of excessive gas and bloating in our gut but more importantly it helps to remove toxins in dried beans. Beans that have been soaked will cook more evenly and quicker. Always discard the soaking water. Then, the next day, when you go to the kitchen to cook, put a big pot of water on the stove and add the drained legumes. Within an hour or two of simmering, they will be ready to cool and store in glass containers in the fridge, ready to use. Cook brown rice, farro or barley too.

Use cooked brown rice or legumes as a side dish for your lunch, or to add to a vegetable soup or stew for dinner. A legume salad with lots of fresh vegetables is a healthy option for lunch or as a side dish for dinner.

COOKING CHICKPEAS

Dried chickpeas triple in size (if not a little more) when cooked, so 220 g (8 oz/1 cup) dried chickpeas will make about 500 g (1 lb 2 oz oz/3 cups) cooked chickpeas.

Add the beans to a large bowl and cover with plenty of water. Soak for 8 hours or overnight. As they rehydrate, the beans absorb the water.

To cook the soaked chickpeas, drain, then add them to a large pot, cover with plenty of water and bring to a boil. Reduce the heat and simmer until they are tender, about 45 minutes to 2 hours, depending on how old the chickpeas are.

When simmering, you can keep the lid off or on but slightly ajar (allowing some steam to escape while cooking so they don't boil over). Chickpeas or beans simmered without a lid will be cooked, but firm. Cooked with the lid on, but ajar, they will be creamier, softer and break apart more easily. These are perfect for hummus or dishes where you want to purée them. Add a generous pinch of salt when they are almost cooked, not at the beginning, as salting the beans too early can cause them to become a little tough.

The cooking time can vary a lot depending on size and freshness, so check them every 30 minutes to judge the best cooking time.

Store the cooked beans in an airtight container in the fridge for up to 5 days, or freeze them for several months.

Once you know how to cook dried chickpeas and beans, you'll always have them on hand. They're really easy to make.

COOKING LENTILS

There's no need to soak lentils, split peas or adzuki beans before you cook them. They can take as little as 20 minutes to cook in water.

Bring plenty of water to a gentle boil, reduce the heat and simmer the lentils for about 30 minutes, discarding any foam that rises to the surface.

COOKING FARRO AND BARLEY

Farro and barley have a chewy texture and nutty flavour. Simply boil water, add the grain and cook until tender.

First, rinse the dried farro or barley in cold water. Bring a pot of water to the boil and add the farro or barley. Cook until it becomes tender and chewy but still has an al dente bite. The cooking time will vary depending on the age and variety of your grain.

When cooked to your liking, drain the grains and run a little cold water through them to stop the cooking. Cooked farro and barley keeps in the fridge for 5 days, but you can freeze it for even longer.

COOKING QUINOA

Quinoa is not actually a grain, but a grain-like seed first grown in South America.

Use 435 ml (15 fl oz/1¾ cups) water for every 200 g (7 oz/1 cup) quinoa. If you use too much water the quinoa can become mushy.

Place the quinoa and water in a medium saucepan and bring to a boil. Cover, then reduce the heat and simmer for 15 minutes. Remove the pan from the heat and let it sit, covered, for another 10 minutes, then remove the lid and fluff up the quinoa with a fork.

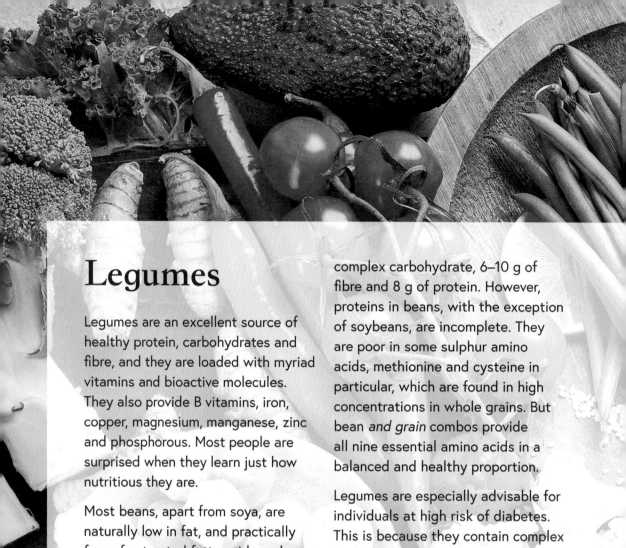

Legumes

Legumes are an excellent source of healthy protein, carbohydrates and fibre, and they are loaded with myriad vitamins and bioactive molecules. They also provide B vitamins, iron, copper, magnesium, manganese, zinc and phosphorous. Most people are surprised when they learn just how nutritious they are.

Most beans, apart from soya, are naturally low in fat, and practically free of saturated fatty acids and cholesterol. One serving of legumes, approximately half a cup, provides on average 120 calories, 20 g of complex carbohydrate, 6–10 g of fibre and 8 g of protein. However, proteins in beans, with the exception of soybeans, are incomplete. They are poor in some sulphur amino acids, methionine and cysteine in particular, which are found in high concentrations in whole grains. But bean *and grain* combos provide all nine essential amino acids in a balanced and healthy proportion.

Legumes are especially advisable for individuals at high risk of diabetes. This is because they contain complex carbohydrates and higher quantities of amylose than most other cereals or tubers, which are slowly digested and have a low glycaemic index.

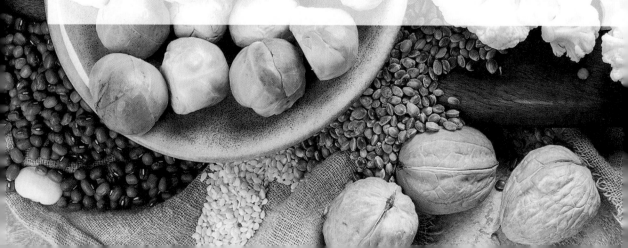

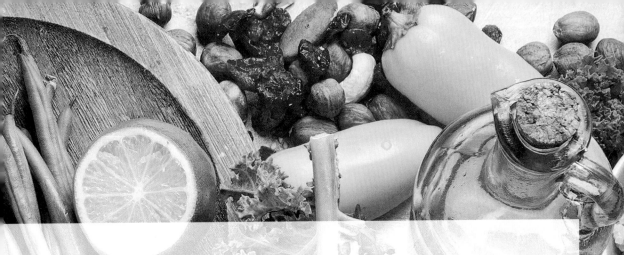

Indeed, legumes do not raise blood glucose and insulin levels as much as other foods with a similar calorie content. A diet rich in legumes may also help with weight control and reducing blood pressure.

Small trials have shown legumes lower blood pressure, independent of weight loss, in people with and without hypertension. By making people feel fuller, the high content of indigestible fibres can promote weight loss.

The fibres also provide a perfect substrate for probiotic bacteria. Some intestinal bacteria that thrive on bean fibre produce a wide range of metabolites that can lower systemic inflammation. Legumes are also one of the best sources of folate, a water-soluble B vitamin essential for creating new red blood cells. This vitamin cannot be stored in our body, which is why we need to consume plenty of folate-rich foods every day, such as legumes, leafy green vegetables, fresh fruits and yeast.

It is true that legumes more than other foods tend to make us produce some extra gas (flatulence), which in some people may cause bloating. Producing gas is a sign that our gut and our microbiome are healthy and working well.

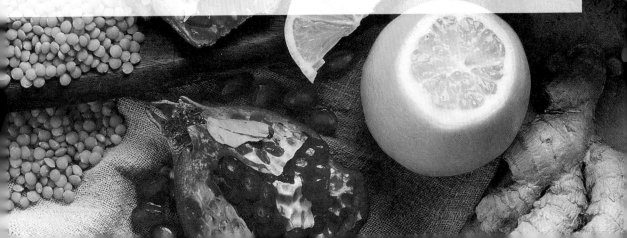

Index

About the authors

Luigi Fontana

Professor Luigi Fontana is a globally recognised physician-scientist and the world's foremost authority in the field of human healthy longevity.

Professor Fontana has worked in some of the world's finest medical institutions, including two that have produced multiple Nobel Laureate, Washington University in St Louis, USA, and the Italian Institute of Health in Rome, Italy. In 2018, Professor Fontana was recruited to the University of Sydney as the Leonard P. Ullmann Chair of Translational Metabolic Health and Director of the Healthy Longevity Research and Clinical Program. He also serves as the Scientific Director of the Charles Perkins Centre Royal Prince Alfred Clinic and the 'Health for Life' Program at the University of Sydney. Additionally, he holds a clinical academic position in the Department of Endocrinology at Royal Prince Alfred Hospital in Sydney, where he continues to practise medicine and conduct groundbreaking research in health, wellbeing, and disease prevention.

Professor Fontana has authored several books and over 160 scientific papers published in esteemed journals, including *Science, Cell, The New England Journal of Medicine, JAMA, BMJ, CA: A Cancer Journal for Clinicians, Nature Reviews Molecular Cell Biology*, and the *European Heart Journal*. He has also delivered over 350 presentations at international conferences and at leading medical schools and research institutes across the globe.

Professor Fontana's contributions to science and medicine have been recognised with numerous prestigious awards. These include the 2009 American Federation for Aging Research (AFAR) Breakthroughs in Gerontology Award, the 2011 Glenn Award for Research in Biological Mechanisms of Aging, the 2016 Vincent Cristofalo Award from AFAR, the 2021 Vice-Chancellor's Award for Excellence from the University of Sydney, and the 2022 Honorary Membership of the Italian Association of Hospital Gastroenterologists. In addition, he has been honoured as an Ordinary Non-Resident Member of both the Italian Academy of Medical and Surgical Sciences of the National Society of Sciences in Naples and the Italian Pontanian Academy of Naples. His leadership roles include serving as a Scientific Member on the Board of Directors of the American Aging Association (2014 – 2019), and since 2016, he has been the Editor-in-Chief of Nutrition and Healthy Aging as well as an Associate Editor of *GeroScience*.

In this book, Professor Fontana distills years of research into practical guidance. He shares evidence-based dietary strategies, whether you are a vegetarian, vegan or omnivore, that you can incorporate into your lifestyle to achieve a longer, healthier and more vibrant life.

Marzio Lanzini

Marzio Lanzini is a multidisciplinary culinary expert with two decades of experience in kitchens across the globe. His expertise encompasses hospitality, food manufacturing, consulting, and project management. As the Healthy Longevity Chef at the Charles Perkins Centre, he runs a cooking program as a part of the CPC RPA Health for Life program, delivering educational programs to schools and patients.

Acknowledgements

This book would not be possible without the love and support of my dear son, Lorenzo, and my mother, Antonietta Iozzi.

There are many others who have inspired and supported me in this amazing journey of discovery. I have also to thank the many postdoctoral fellows, PhD students and medical students who were critical to my lab's success.

In particular, I would like to thank and acknowledge the help of Marzio Lanzini, who tested and photographed all the recipes for this book in the metabolic kitchen that was established to show patients, students and others better ways to eat.

A special thank you goes to my publisher, Pam Brewster, who helped to craft this practical book that complements my previous books, *The Path to Longevity* and *Manual of Healthy Longevity and Wellbeing*.

Published in 2025 by Hardie Grant Books, an imprint of Hardie Grant Publishing

Hardie Grant Books (Melbourne)
Wurundjeri Country
Building 1, 658 Church Street
Richmond, Victoria 3121

Hardie Grant North America
2912 Telegraph Ave
Berkeley, California 94705

hardiegrant.com/books

Hardie Grant acknowledges the Traditional Owners of the Country on which we work, the Wurundjeri People of the Kulin Nation and the Gadigal People of the Eora Nation, and recognises their continuing connection to the land, waters and culture. We pay our respects to their Elders past and present.

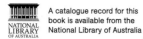

A catalogue record for this book is available from the National Library of Australia

Plant Power

ISBN 978 1 76145 088 4
ISBN 978 1 76144 213 1 (ebook)

10 9 8 7 6 5 4 3 2 1

Publishing Director: Pam Brewster
Head of Editorial: Jasmin Chua
Project Editor: Lauren Carta
Editor: Kate Daniel
Designer: Alicia May
Additional photography: istock
Typesetting: Hannah Schubert
Head of Production: Todd Rechner
Production Controller: Jessica Harvie

Colour reproduction by Splitting Image Colour Studio

Printed in China by Leo Paper Products LTD.

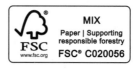